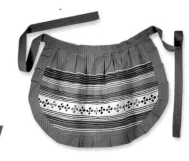

Aprons
of the Mid-20th Century

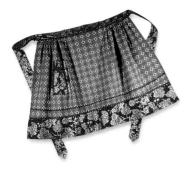

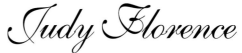

Judy Florence

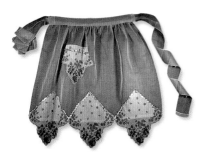

To Serve and Protect

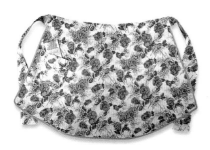

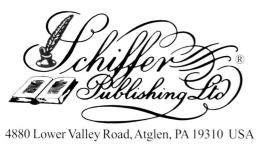

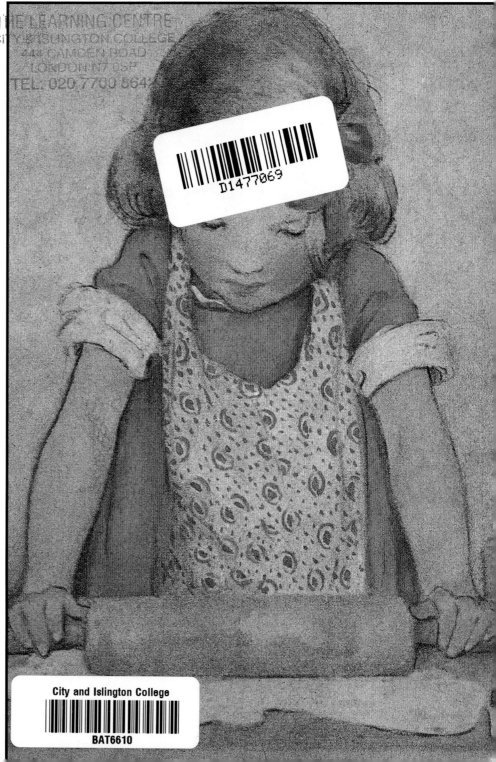

Schiffer Publishing Ltd

4880 Lower Valley Road, Atglen, PA 19310 USA

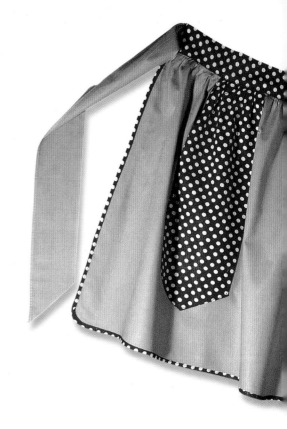

Dedication

To my mother, Eilene Paulson, and my sister, Jean Paulson, who always wore aprons, and still do.

Credits

All apron photographs by Jim Simonsen, unless otherwise specified.

All aprons from the collection of the author, unless otherwise specified.

Cover image from *Electric Cooking with your Hotpoint Automatic Range*, ©Hotpoint Institute

Designed by Bonnie M. Hensley
Cover design by Bruce M. Waters
Type set in Bernhard Mod BT/Humanist 521 BT

ISBN: 0-7643-1341-X
Printed in China
1 2 3 4

Published by Schiffer Publishing Ltd.
4880 Lower Valley Road
Atglen, PA 19310
Phone: (610) 593-1777; Fax: (610) 593-2002
E-mail: Schifferbk@aol.com
Please visit our web site catalog at
www.schifferbooks.com

This book may be purchased from the publisher.
Include $3.95 for shipping. Please try your bookstore first.
We are always looking for people to write books on new and related subjects. If you have an idea for a book please contact us at the above address.
You may write for a free catalog.

In Europe, Schiffer books are distributed by
Bushwood Books
6 Marksbury Avenue
Kew Gardens
Surrey TW9 4JF England
Phone: 44 (0) 20-8392-8585; Fax: 44 (0) 20-8392-9876
E-mail: Bushwd@aol.com
Free postage in the UK. Europe: air mail at cost.

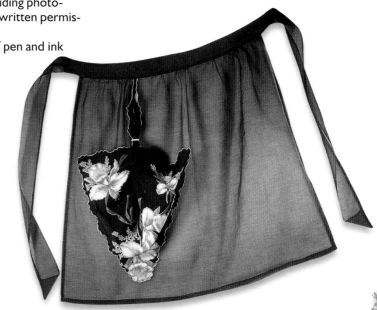

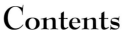

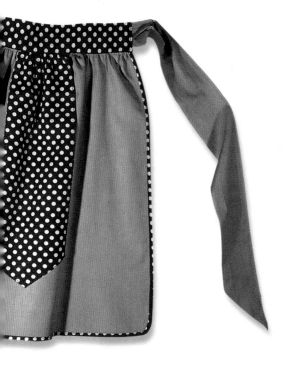

Contents

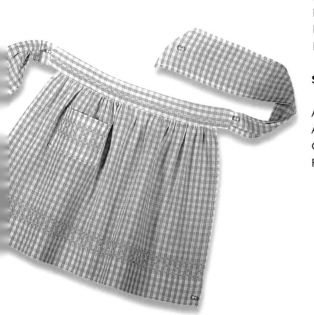

Preface

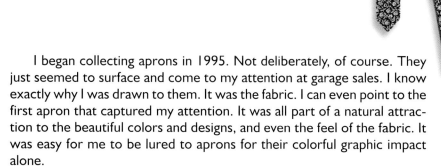

I began collecting aprons in 1995. Not deliberately, of course. They just seemed to surface and come to my attention at garage sales. I know exactly why I was drawn to them. It was the fabric. I can even point to the first apron that captured my attention. It was all part of a natural attraction to the beautiful colors and designs, and even the feel of the fabric. It was easy for me to be lured to aprons for their colorful graphic impact alone.

This should not have been a surprise to me, as I have been actively participating and circulating in the world of quiltmaking for over thirty years. The very essence of quiltmaking is fabric. If you have ever visited one of the quilt exhibitions or fabric shops that have popped up across the country (and indeed, around the world) in the last quarter century, you know what I mean. They literally overflow with fabric and color. Most of my adult life has been immersed in quilt-related activities—finding fabrics, coordinating and contrasting colors, modifying designs, even dyeing some of my own fabrics. This natural affinity for fabric has carried over to additional textiles. Aprons just happen to be the area which got the first stronghold in my new ventures into other fiber arts and household linens.

Each time I brought home a newly discovered apron from yet another neighborhood thrift sale, I would show it to my closest quiltmaking friends. They derived a good deal of pleasure in seeing these beautiful fabrics, too. It was not very long, of course, before the inevitable question was raised. Was I collecting aprons? Certainly not, was the answer. I just brought them home because the fabrics were quite unusual and oh-so-gorgeous, unlike anything else in my (or their) collections, unlike anything you would be able to find in a fabric store these days.

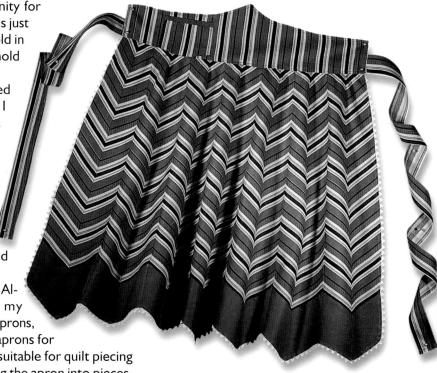

A note of clarification must be made here. Although it was my fondness for fabric and my quiltmaking background that drew me toward the aprons, I never *seriously* considered using fabric from the aprons for my quilts. Many of the apron fabrics are perfectly suitable for quilt piecing or appliqué, but I totally rejected the idea of cutting the apron into pieces. This was evidence to me that it was not only the *fabric* that I treasured. I also valued the apron for its *design*, perhaps even for its purpose and its past.

You can probably predict the rest of the story. One apron became a few, a few became many, and many became a substantial stack in the closet. It was then I realized I truly was collecting aprons. From that point on my efforts in seeking out and gathering aprons to round out my collection were more concerted.

I didn't need or rely on encouragement from anyone else. Going to garage sales was already one of my favored pastimes. I just became more aware of the growing number of household textiles and linens that were available, especially aprons. Many were in very good or excellent condition, and most were reasonably priced. I was dedicated to gathering the most unusual and impressive apron designs and making minor reparations to those that required it. Laundering, stain removal, ironing, and mending of seams, sashes, and tears became a routine task following a garage sale or flea market jaunt.

Eventually I began to regard my apron collection more seriously. When the number and variety became quite significant, I decided to study them more thoroughly. As I inspected them, I made written notes about the unique features of each apron, and I compared and contrasted their details. The amount of detail found on a single apron surprised me. At first it seemed like either quite insignificant or overly obvious stuff, e.g., 'apron has rickrack trim' (which might be just like a hundred other aprons). Except *this* apron had 'rickrack trim in two sizes, one with gold metallic thread, and applied in unusual parallel rows on the waistband.' Or 'apron has embroidery.' Except *this* apron had 'Swedish *huck* embroidery on a six inch border, worked in double stranded floss in three shades of pink.' It became clear to me there was more to my collection than 'just a bunch of aprons,' perhaps something worthy of study and preservation.

Thus began my focused effort to document my apron collection. Additional visits to garage sales, flea markets, and antique malls were scheduled, and my storage containers began to bulge. My once-thin file folders of research notations began to acquire heft.

When participants were asked to introduce themselves at a recent class that I attended, I identified myself as a textile conservator (the first time I had said it *out loud*, to a group of people I barely knew). I was pleasantly surprised by their response—a mixture of intrigue and respect, followed by sincere questions. Up until that time I had jokingly referred to myself as a textile conservator, mainly to the members of my immediate family, in an attempt to infuse some credibility into what I was doing. It sounded rather lofty to me, but I felt it accurately described what I was doing. A conservator is 'one that preserves from injury or violation.' I believed I was protecting and preserving aprons from their possible misuse or even disposal or destruction.

That minor but memorable experience helped me understand I really am a textile conservator, or at least an *emerging* textile conservator. The list of textiles I have been gathering and conserving is assorted and quite long. Aprons are currently at the top.

Judy Florence
Textile Conservator

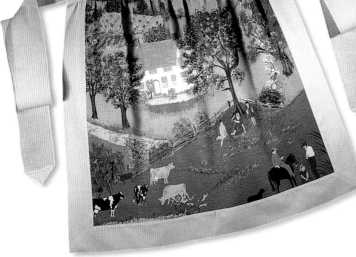

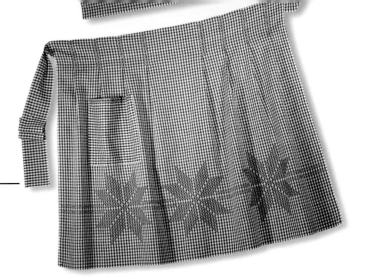

Acknowledgments

Many people have been very helpful during the preparation and writing of this book. Some in small ways, others in large. I am grateful for their cooperation and generosity in sharing aprons, information, references, photographs, personal stories, ideas, opinions, time, and advice.

Thanks to my mother, Eilene Paulson, and my sister Jean Paulson. Others who eagerly made contributions are Arda Davis, Janet Carson, Pat Simonsen, Betty Wilson, Lucy Bauer, Cindy Paulson, Vivian Mets, and Virginia Bregel. Thanks to the South Shore Quilters of Cornucopia, Wisconsin who cheerfully participated in my initial research.

I appreciate the willingness of contemporary artist Christine Ilewski from Alton, Illinois to share her artwork and photographs. The proprietors of several vintage linen and antique shops have also assisted me: Kim Schiller of *Thode's Mercantile* in Augusta, Wisconsin, Terri Wyman of *The Hedgehog* in Cornucopia, Wisconsin, and Sue Loomer of *Grand Remnants* in St. Paul, Minnesota.

As always, my husband Dick and our sons Matt and Dave displayed an extraordinary amount of patience and encouragement when I most needed it.

I am particularly indebted to Jim Simonsen for the creation of this book. He is a talented photographer and longtime family friend. It was with his generosity and sense of adventure that this book was made possible and the project was made pleasurable.

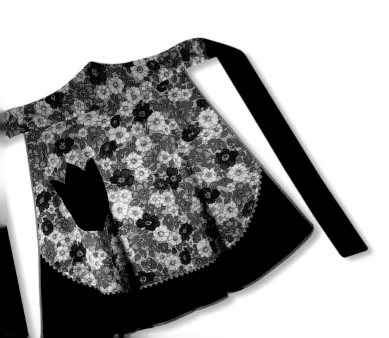

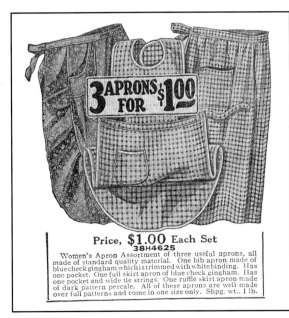

Aprons from the 1922 Sears Catalog, page 146,
©Sears, Roebuck and Co.

"3 Aprons for $1.00," 1922 Sears Catalog, page 146,
©Sears, Roebuck and Co.

Introduction

An Indispensable Part of the Wardrobe

In the world of textiles and household linens, aprons have been largely ignored. Mostly regarded as useless relics of the past, many have made their way to the back of the linen closet or the bottom of the kitchen drawer. Others have been disposed of, their useful life at an end. A few treasured aprons have been tucked away in cedar chests.

In past generations, aprons were an indispensable part of a woman's (and sometimes a man's) wardrobe. Special aprons were designed for specific household tasks. They were not simply for meal preparation and serving tea to guests. Examples of everyday tasks for which an apron was worn included washing clothes, washing hair, dusting and household pickup, vacuuming, nursing a baby, feeding an infant, bathing a baby, home nursing, preparing food, preserving food, serving guests, gathering garden produce, gathering flowers, knitting (and other needlework), dressmaking, mending, hanging out laundry, carrying wood, painting, and varnishing.

The 1922 Sears Catalog pictures and describes several apron styles, most of them in a full style that covers the entire front of the body, worn by women in stylish dresses and high-heeled shoes. Featured top and center on page 146 is a set of "3 aprons for $1.00." The description reads:

> Women's Apron Assortment of three useful aprons all made of standard quality material. One bib apron made of blue check gingham which is trimmed with white binding. Has one pocket. One full skirt apron of blue check gingham. Has one pocket and wide tie strings. One ruffle skirt apron made of dark pattern percale. All of these aprons are well made over full patterns and come in one size only.

The 1922 Sears Catalog also has several photos of women attired in aprons, and it's not the *apron* that is being described and marketed. Aproned women are prominently included in advertisements for washing machines, hot water heating systems, irons, bathroom fixtures, paint, and dinnerware. The woman on page 725 is poised at the edge of a bathtub, helping a child wash her hair. The picture features the sink and tub of the newfangled Iroquois Bathroom Outfit. Properly attired and neatly coifed, it's as if the woman would be less-than-dressed if she were not wearing an apron.

The 1935-36 Fall/Winter Sears Catalog has several pages of women's aprons. "Gay Border Print Anchor-Back Aprons" are shown on page 71. They are described as "Washfast Percale, Perfect Gifts, Real Sears Value, Assorted Colorful Prints, a Set of 2 for 49¢."

Somewhat higher quality "Gay Coverall Aprons in Assorted Border Prints" are found on page 82. The description reads: "Attractive, Practical, Anchor Back aprons won't roll or ride up! Washfast, Printed Percale with piping trim," and the price is 39¢ each or 2 for 75¢.

And if you choose to sew your own apron, suitable percale can be found on page 395 of the same 1935-36 catalog. The advertisement features a woman in a full-length apron. Available in 36-inch widths, the fabric is billed as washfast and boilfast, in brand new styles:

Percales fast to washing and boiling almost always cost more than this price! And especially when the prints are as pretty and smart as these. Good serviceable quality.

Pages full of aprons can still be found in the catalogs of the 1940s. The 1942-43 Fall/Winter Montgomery Ward Catalog pictures many styles modeled by happy housewives. Smocks and coverall styles prevail on page 125. In addition, companion mother/daughter styles are featured. Displayed across the center of the page is the bargain "Box of Three Aprons for $1.29."

Box of 3 aprons at right...consists of one green striped apron, one assorted floral pattern, and one Copen Blue polka dot apron. They are all in washable percale. The box of 3 is an ideal and practical gift—one everyone would love to receive. Each apron is bias bound and the polka dot apron has rickrack trim in addition to the bias. One size fits 30-38" bust.

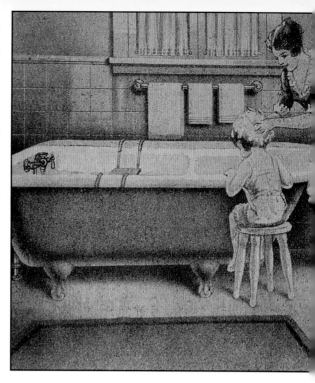

The woman on page 1062 of the same catalog wears a protective full style apron while varnishing her floor. Similarly aproned women can be found on nearby pages promoting sundry home improvement and cleaning products.

It's clear that aprons weren't confined to the kitchen. In the *Home Laundering Guide for Clothes and Fabrics* published by the Westinghouse Home Economics Institute in 1944, a woman is pictured doing laundry in a wringer washing machine, washing clothes by hand in a laundry tub, and ironing clothes. In each instance, she is wearing a stylish bibbed apron with shoulder ruffles, drop down waist, patch pockets, and decorative edging.

In the 1954 *Simplicity Sewing Book: Easy Guide for Beginners and Experts* a woman and a girl are featured on the front cover. The woman is smartly outfitted in an over-the-shoulder and around-the-back red and white striped apron.

The cover of the pamphlet *How to Sew and Save with Cotton Bags* features a smiling woman in her feed sack apron. It is a bibbed design made from plaid fabric, with ruffled edging and a giant bow at the back. The woman is happily making preparations for use of another cotton bag. A suitable pattern for a bibbed and buttoned full length apron (#8136) is casually modeled by a slender and short-haired lady.

The attractive woman on the cover of Hamilton Beach's Mixette *Recipe and Instruction Book* is somewhere in the vicinity of the kitchen. In addition to being glowingly made up and smartly dressed, she sports a very showy bibbed and sashed apron made from a bold floral print with contrasting waistband and shoulder panels.

Magazine articles and advertisements often depicted women in aprons, especially with kitchen and food related subjects. The familiar traditional Thanksgiving holiday scene with the husband and wife, 2.3 children, and great grandmother seated at the dining room table, anxiously awaiting the carving of the roasted turkey by grandfather and delivery of the cranber-

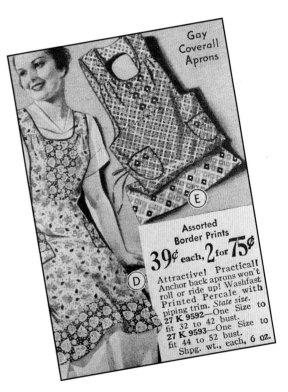

"Gay Coverall Aprons," 1935-36 Fall/Winter Sears Catalog, page 82, ©Sears, Roebuck and Co.

Box of Three Aprons at right—the box consists of one green striped apron—one assorted floral pattern apron and one Copen Blue polka dot apron. They are all in washable percale. The box of three is an ideal and practical gift—one everyone would love to receive. Each apron is bias bound and the polka dot has rickrack trim in addition to the binding. One size — fits 30 to 38-inch bust. Ship. wt. 1 lb.
15 C 1129—Box of three aprons..................$1.29

Include all your little house dresses in your budget. It is so convenient to buy on time. For complete details of Time Payment Plan see the Inside Back Cover.

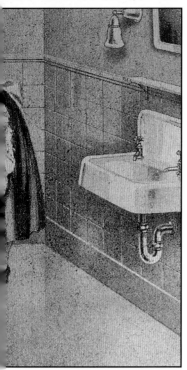

Mother wearing apron while bathing a child; advertisement for Iroquois Bathroom Outfit, 1922 Sears Catalog, p. 725, ©Sears, Roebuck and Co.

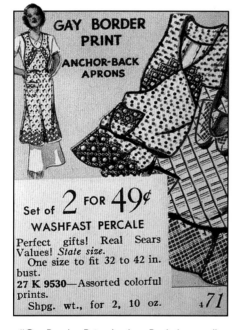

"Gay Border Print Anchor-Back Aprons," 1935-36 Fall/Winter Sears Catalog, page 71, ©Sears, Roebuck and Co.

"Box of Three Aprons for $1.29," 1942-43 Fall/Winter Montgomery Ward Catalog, page 125, ©Montgomery Ward

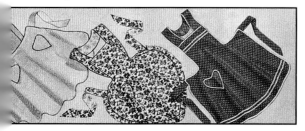

ries and relishes by the apron-clad grandmother has appeared in various versions in countless serial publications and calendars.

The husband, son, and daughter appear equally anxious for the arrival of the roasted turkey in the cover photo of *Electric Cooking with your Hotpoint Automatic Range*. And so mother once again delivers the goods, proudly outfitted in her neatly ruffled and sashed apron.

Although I can guarantee that our family Thanksgiving gatherings do not look exactly like that, I do have evidence of similar scenarios in my family's history. The black and white Thanksgiving photograph is a 1936 gathering of my paternal grandmother and several of my aunts, uncles, and cousins (and the dog). The roasted bird is positioned prominently on a serving cart at front left. The table is set formally, the guests dressed properly. And my Aunt Nelle is wearing her *good* apron with the rickrack edging, having likely just changed from her *everyday* kitchen apron.

Getting Personal

On a more familiar level, my experience with aprons dates back to around 1950. As a child, I wore aprons sewn by my mother for my sister and me, two of which are included in the *Children's Aprons* section of this book. One is a smock style with a back button closure and three generous pockets. It is made from blue cotton fabric that remains familiar to me because I also have a 1950s vintage housecoat that my mother cut from the same cloth.

The other child's apron is a pinafore style made from blue printed gingham checked cloth with a bib, shoulder straps, and red rickrack trim. It, too, was used by my sister and me. As a youngster growing up on a family farm, I was very active in food preparation and preservation. Although I don't remember wearing particular aprons, I know that I did wear them. And if I didn't, I was frequently reminded by my mother to do so.

Like tens of thousands of teenage girls across America, the first apron I made was in a high school home economics class. I still have the apron and the original pattern. That was during my freshman year, 1959-60. It was a cobbler style pattern (Advance #7878), price 25 cents. I split the cost and shared the pattern with another girl, whose name is also penciled on the front of the pattern.

The apron featured large pockets along the lower edge, tie ends that were sewn into the darts, and bias trim around the armholes, neckline, pockets, and back closing edges. It was clearly a practical and protective design. I don't recall using the apron much during my high school years except when required during cooking classes. It surfaced many years later, and can still be found in my kitchen drawer. When I feel like I *really* need protection I wear this apron, which is designed to accommodate major dribbles and splatters.

The second apron I made was part of a 4-H clothing construction project. I have the details for a cross stitched gingham apron in my 1961 4-H record book. The sample swatch is still glued in place for a pink apron with pocket, sashes, and brown cross stitching. It took four hours to complete and cost 63 cents to make. (I checked fabric prices in an early 1960s Sears catalog, and yes, gingham was 64 cents a yard.) I made the apron as part of a project to sew clothes for several family members. The apron was for my grandmother. I completed it on 12-23-61, just in time to give it to her for Christmas.

It was thirty years before I made another apron. In the 1990s I made three more, each created specifically for periodical publication. All three were original quilted designs. Two were made from recycled cotton bags, one from a flour sack, the other from a rice sack.

Portions of a 25-pound Stockton Roller Mill natural unbleached flour sack are used in the rounded bib and pocket of the blue apron pictured here. Thick waistline gathers and a ruffled lower edge define the long skirt. The bib and pocket are hand quilted and the apron is machine stitched.

My kitchen drawer has a few aprons in it. My current favorite is made from a recycled unbleached muslin rice sack. It was made by a friend. It is a simple one-piece style with extra long bright pink ties that loop behind the neck and around the waist. The words *Kokuho Rose* appear boldly across the bodice, along with Chinese characters, Japanese lettering, and English information. Most importantly, it has two huge pockets. It is sadly faded from intensive use and repeated launderings over the years, and my family thinks it looks quite awful, but I cherish it greatly.

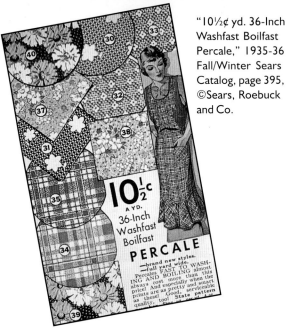

"10½¢ yd. 36-Inch Washfast Boilfast Percale," 1935-36 Fall/Winter Sears Catalog, page 395, ©Sears, Roebuck and Co.

An Informal Research Method

When I began to examine the aprons in my collection more thoroughly, I discovered many previously unnoticed details. My self-designed system for 'documentation' was quite simple. First I checked each apron for needed repairs and stains. (I had previously washed all the aprons.) After minor sewing reparations and stain removal (rarely required), I sprinkled and steam pressed each apron, folded it in half lengthwise, and hung it on a wooden pants hanger.

The next step involved observation of details. I usually began this as I ironed each apron, a pencil and notebook at the ready, jotting down what I considered important information. I also listed not-so-important information. Some of the specifics included:

- overall style
- general condition
- dimensions
- fiber content
- type of fabric
- colors
- construction techniques
- date made
- where it was made
- who made it
- who wore it
- embellishments
- pocket style
- sash style
- waistband style
- labels
- source
- date of acquisition
- cost

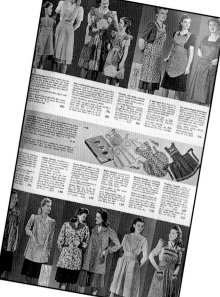

Aprons from the 1942-43 Fall/Winter Montgomery Ward Catalog, page 125, ©Montgomery Ward

Not all of these categories would apply to a given apron. Some information was either unavailable or not applicable. There was plenty to be noted about some aprons; others seemed undistinguished, and I had to really search for anything noteworthy and for features that set them apart from the others.

By this point I had chosen to limit my research to the half aprons in my collection. For the purposes of this project, all the others were set aside. I eliminated smocks, coveralls, bibbed, crocheted, and other specialty designs. The *overall style* of all the aprons is *half* apron. Nearly all of them have a skirt, a waistband, sashes, and perhaps a pocket. Other overall

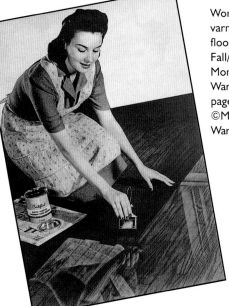

Woman in apron varnishing the floor, 1942-43 Fall/Winter Montgomery Ward Catalog, page 1062, ©Montgomery Ward

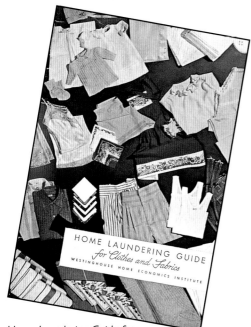

Home Laundering Guide for Clothes and Fabrics, Westinghouse Home Economics Institute, ©1944, Westinghouse Electric & Mfg. Co.

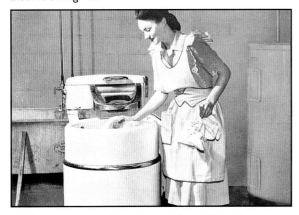

Woman in apron doing the weekly washing, *Home Laundering Guide for Clothes and Fabrics*, page 9, ©1944, Westinghouse Electric & Mfg. Co.

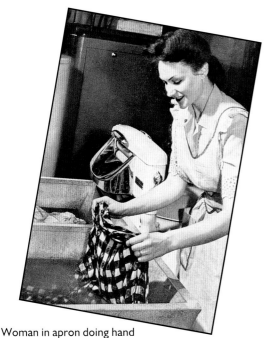

Woman in apron doing hand laundry, *Home Laundering Guide for Clothes and Fabrics*, page 20, ©1944, Westinghouse Electric and Mfg. Co.

style details include aprons with overskirts, gored aprons, and reversible patterns.

The *general condition* didn't vary a great deal from one apron to the next. If it wasn't in good condition to begin with, I probably left it on the garage sale table or in the vendor's display. If it was *entirely* new, this was noted. For some aprons, the indicators of use and wear were listed. This might be an overall look or feel of wearing thin. Also any lingering stains and evidence of repair work, e.g., patches over holes, restitching on pocket corners or sashes. Color fading was ascertained by comparing the right side of the fabric on the *outside* of the apron with the right side of the fabric on the *inside*.

Indicators of *non*-use are details such as entirely intact 'pinked' seams and still visible markings for prestamped embroidery patterns. Indicators of *use* include unyielding wrinkles (especially on cotton), stress marks on the sashes (especially on organdy), fraying of seams, and raveling of edges. Also a lifetime supply of lint in the pockets and pointed sash ends.

Apron *dimensions* were noted only if they were out of the ordinary, e.g., unusually small or large, disproportionate, odd shaped. Dimensional notes were made more frequently for children's aprons, in order to accurately visualize them and distinguish them from adult aprons.

The *fiber content* was not always easy to identify. Most are cotton or linen (natural fibers), a few are nylon, acetate, rayon, or polyester (synthetic fibers), and even fewer are blends. Tidbits from a textile chemistry course were excavated from the recesses of my mind, and textile handbooks were consulted. Because the overwhelming majority are cotton, the fiber content is not always noted in the captions.

Common *types of fabric* include muslin, percale, batiste, lawn, broadcloth, gingham, organdy, dotted Swiss, organza, tulle, and taffeta. Descriptions of these fabrics are located in the *Glossary* at the back of the book. Cotton percale, gingham, and organdy appear most frequently. Other types of fabrics noted were recycled cotton bags, cotton towels, huck toweling, decorator cloth, shirting, polished cotton, flocked cloth, and handkerchiefs.

Colors were specified not only because of their visual effects, but also to assist in dating. Certain colors can be associated with certain eras, e.g., turquoise with the 1950s. I used colors to organize some sections of the book: Gingham aprons were selected and grouped by their range of colors (*Every Color Under the Sun*), and the *Color Gallery* section highlights designs in Red, Pink, Yellow, and Purple.

Construction techniques comprises many things. First, was it made by hand or machine, or a combination? Hand stitching can be distinguished from machine stitching fairly easily. Distinguishing 'home made' from 'store bought' (factory made) is not so easy. A store-bought apron could be combined with handwork done at home, e.g., a prestamped embroidery kit. Aprons made in the home usually combined both hand and machine stitching. Aprons made in the factory rarely included hand stitching. An *entirely* hand sewn apron is a delight to find and a wonder to behold.

Other construction details noted were the types of stitching—straight, zigzag, buttonhole, etc. Special embroidery stitches were recorded with information about embellishments. Methods of gathering, pleating, and ruffling were recorded and sketches and measurements were taken.

The history of an apron is more elusive. Unless the maker or owner are available for questioning, the *date made, where it was made, who made it, and who wore it* usually remain a mystery. But when such information is available, it can be the most intimate and intriguing portion of the data. Aprons from antique stores and flea markets rarely carry a pedigree. Those from garage sales have a better chance of carrying personal details. Aprons from one's family or friends usually abound with morsels of a private nature.

Some of the examples pictured in the book came directly from the cedar chest or closet of a friend or family member. These are the ones with stories to tell. Frankly, I assign greater value to the familial history of an apron than to its birth date. Precision dating and longevity are impressive and important, but the personal account has more appeal for me.

Embellishments are such a significant factor in apron design that several sections of the book are devoted to them. Adornments such as rickrack, needle arts, and piecing and appliqué are examined. Rickrack is a study in itself. Details of colors, styles, sizes, and methods of application are discussed and shown in the section *When Rickrack was the Rage*. However, because rickrack was so universally popular among apron makers, good examples appear in every section of the book.

Needle art details include embroidery, crocheting, tatting, and lace. Embroidery was examined to determine if it was hand or machine worked. Patterns, colors, and types of embroidery stitches were also noted. Many aprons boasted decorative edgings and inserts of crochet, lace, and tatting. Examples are pictured in the *Needle Arts* section.

Many aprons are embellished with piecing and appliqué. These quilt-related techniques can be by hand or machine, intricate or bold. Aprons so adorned are shown in the *Pieced and Appliquéd* chapter.

I was in for a pleasant surprise when I considered *pocket styles*. Sketches of different shapes were made as I studied each apron. The variety was substantial. What is traditionally available in a choice of square or rounded, was found in dozens of arrangements: triangular, square, rectangular, pentagonal, hexagonal, free form, rounded, stylized. Pockets were shaped like objects—hearts, mittens, flowers. Check the *A Pocket for Every Purpose* section for particulars.

Sash and waistband styles are not limited to long and rectangular. In addition to differences in length and width, many waistbands are shaped with graceful upper and lower curves, some heart shaped. Others have zigzag or notched upper edges or drop down V-shaped lower edges. Still others are embellished with bias trim, rickrack or embroidery.

Sash widths vary greatly—from very narrow (half inch) to extremely wide (five inches). Similarly, the hems at the ends of the sashes vary from an eighth of an inch to three inches deep. The ends might be square, triangular, pointed, or curved; and they are a potential site for rickrack, cross stitch, embroidery, and lace.

And what *labels* might be found? Perhaps a commercial label, concrete evidence that the apron was factory made. Or maybe a personal label, which might take the form of an embroidered or cross stitched name or initials, an attached cloth tag inscribed with one's name, or marking with an indelible pen or marker. Labels are more the exception than the rule on aprons.

If known, the specific *source, date of acquisition, and cost* were recorded. All too often, this information was either not available or I didn't have the foresight to write it down at the time of purchase or receipt. I can generally recall if an apron was purchased at a garage sale, thrift store, or antique store. Or if it was given to me, and by whom. But I'm less likely to remember when or in which shop (maybe the city or state). As I became more serious about my research, I also grew more vigilant about recording these details.

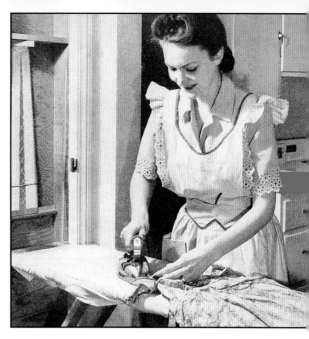

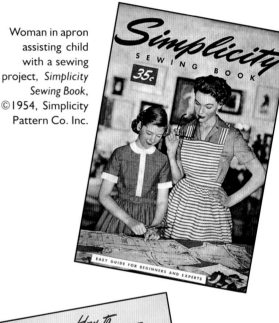

Woman in apron assisting child with a sewing project, *Simplicity Sewing Book*, ©1954, Simplicity Pattern Co. Inc.

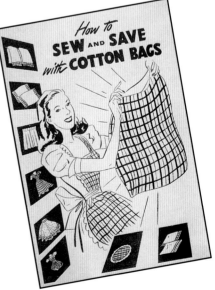

Woman preparing a cotton bag for a sewing project, *How to Sew and Save with Cotton Bags*, ©National Cotton Council

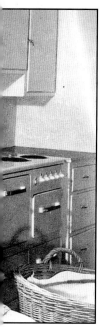

Woman in apron ironing the weekly wash, *Home Laundering Guide for Clothes and Fabrics*, page 26, ©1944, Westinghouse Electric & Mfg. Co.

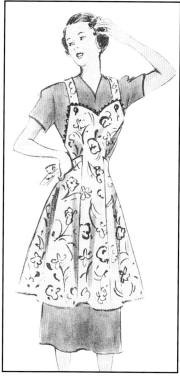

Apron pattern #8136 using recycled cotton bags, *How to Sew and Save with Cotton Bags*, ©National Cotton Council

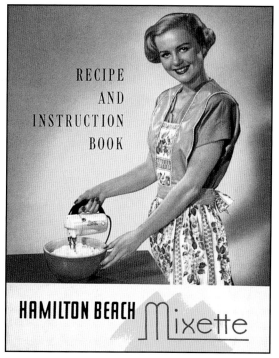

Woman in apron preparing food with electric mixer, *Recipe and Instruction Book*, ©Hamilton Beach Company

Men in Aprons

The 1922 Sears catalog pictures several men in aprons, each seriously attired in preparation for work. Assorted apron styles could be ordered. They were all job-related, each generously cut and obviously designed for protection. *Maximum* protection.

Men in aprons are historically associated with occupations I have dubbed 'the three B's': blacksmith, butcher, and baker. To that list of B's we can add men in their more contemporary callings as bartenders and barbecue chefs. Together those five occupations encompass a vast majority of the men who wear or wore aprons. Catalogs from the first half of the 20th century also picture men's aprons for dairy and milking chores, picking fruits and vegetables, carpentry (leather aprons), and mechanics.

The black and white photograph of the men in their overalls and the cook in his bibbed apron is a nostalgic pictorial commentary on occupations and attire. A hat, a shirt, and bibbed overalls are standard costume for most of the men. One is dressed more formally with dress pants, necktie, and cardigan, and one gentleman tops his overalls with a suit jacket. The cook stands out prominently, bare-headed, hands on his hips, proudly sporting an extra long white bibbed apron. He is the visual focus of the picture, if not the center of attention in the group. His purely protective and functional apron proclaims his occupation and status, loudly and clearly.

All the associations of men and aprons I found had to do with aprons as utilitarian garments, as protective shields. All were work related. None were decorative. In a man's world, aprons are serious business.

Children in Aprons

Many cookbooks published specifically for children include photographs of girls (and some boys) in aprons. Pictures from three cookbooks, published in 1932, 1955, and 1957 are shown here.

The young lass on the cover of *Kitchen Fun: A Cook Book for Children* wears a ribbon bow in her hair and a loosely hung apron of printed material around her neck. With ingredients and utensils at hand, she is clearly focused on her task of rolling out some sort of doughy mass. She has followed the second rule from the *Rules for Little Cooks*—PUT ON YOUR APRON. (Second only to the first rule, which is *Wash your hands*). This was good advice from the Harter Publishing Company in 1932, and it's equally good advice today.

The young lady seated on the blue hassock has progressed to the third rule—*Read your recipe carefully*. She has already donned her widely-flared pinafore-style apron with its long sashes and large bow and is perusing her recipe.

The girls in the 1955 *Mary Alden's Cookbook for Children* also favor pinafore style aprons. The smiling young lady on the cover is wearing a ruffled and sashed ash gray apron while stirring the cookie dough. The girl cutting the cooled brownies wears a white bibbed apron with colorful trim down the front and across the patch pocket. The pig-tailed girl making her delivery of steaming hot franks and beans is also outfitted in a stylish white pinafore apron with red decoration.

In the 1957 *Betty Crocker's Cook Book for Boys and Girls* several children are shown preparing and serving food. Boys and girls alike are illustrated with aprons of various styles. On the cover is a young girl with an egg beater in her hands and a pink bibbed and sashed apron over her clothes. Mother, too, is properly outfitted in her blue gathered half apron.

Mother and daughter combination patterns were also popular throughout the 20th century. Ready-made aprons and patterns for home sewing were available from mail order catalogs. The pictured "Me and Ma" apron pattern "consisting of identical designs for mother and child" was published in 1925 by The Pictorial Review Company, New York. The 1942-43 Fall/Winter Montgomery Ward Catalog pictured mothers and daughters in look alike bibbed and pinafored aprons, described as follows:

> Mother and Daughter apron set in better quality tubfast percale. Rickrack trims the two large pockets, the bib, straps, and edges the entire apron. It's such fun to dress alike that mother will have no trouble at all getting help around the house.
>
> Gay multicolorful patchwork pattern pinafore apron—it will fit all sizes—for mother and daughter. Two huge roomy pockets—very full skirt on a set-in waistband. Deep ruffles over the shoulders extend from the front waist to the back waistband. In washable cotton print.

The pages of the 1937 *Elson Pupil's Hand Chart* are strewn with drawings of both mothers and girls in aprons. Mother is wearing an apron while she waters the flowers, mends the family's clothes, bakes cookies, knits, and feeds the animals. The young girl wears a coverall style apron over her dress during indoor play, outdoor play, gardening, and with her pets. A child's coverall style apron very similar to the one in the Elson book is included in the *Children's Aprons* section of this book.

Their distinctive connection with cherished childhood memories make children's aprons an especially alluring topic. A special section of this book is devoted exclusively to them. Seventeen aprons in a variety of styles are pictured and described. Companion mother/daughter designs are also included. Patterns for children's aprons are shown in the *Appendix: An Assortment of Vintage Apron Patterns and Kits*.

Aprons And Domesticity:
A Contemporary View

The association of aprons with domesticity has been explored by several contemporary visual artists. Christine Ilewski included aprons as part of her 1988 Bachelor of Fine Arts exhibition. In a combination of silk screening and painting, images from her personal, family, maternal, and religious life were graphically portrayed on traditional aprons. Each apron had its "story" written on it. Some details were hand-painted, others inscribed or drawn onto the surface of the fabric.

Ms. Ilewski states that her aprons were about women's history of domesticity and its limitations. Marriage and divorce, Catholicism, and the birthing and raising of a child are the heavy duty subjects of her works. She silk screened directly on cotton aprons in graphic images. She presents her serious and thought-provoking subject matter in a graphic format, in unquestionable rebellion to the domesticity and restrictions associated with women's aprons.

Christine's first apron pictures three old ladies looking through a window at a younger woman. The words read "I'd take the streetcar downtown to do my shopping. We'd get on, the baby in my arms, Gary holding onto my skirt, and Gail holding the diaper bag. I'd see those old ladies staring at us from across the aisle, looking at me like 'you poor thing' and I'd think to myself, 'I'm not doing so bad.'" This is based on her grandmother's memories of being a young mother during the Depression in St. Louis.

Apron-clad mother delivering the roasted turkey, *Electric Cooking with your Hotpoint Automatic Range*, ©Hotpoint Institute

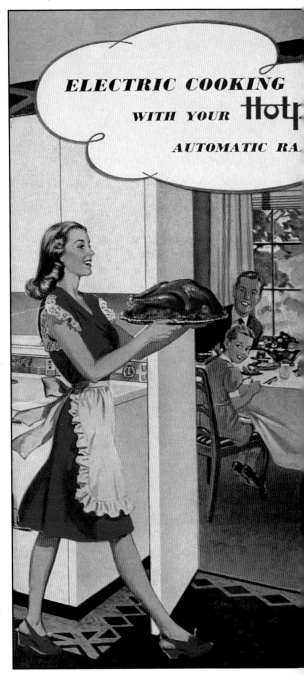

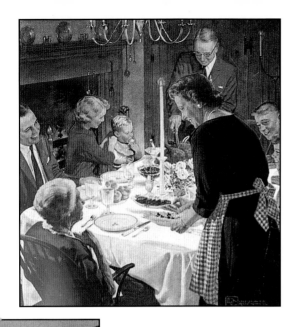

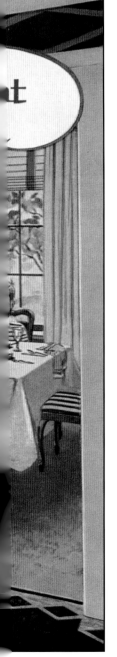

The red half apron has an old Catholic church, a child's face cradled in two hands, and two small photos of the faces of Christine and her father collaged over graphic dancers' faces. The text reads, "As a little girl my father would take me to church. He'd sit me down in the front pew and speak to me from the lectern. His voice hung on the words of Matthew, Mark, Luke, and John. He spoke of love and responsibility. He said that he was responsible for me, for my heart, my mind, and my soul." This apron design is based on Sundays Christine spent going to Catholic mass with her father, his strong Polish heritage, and the words he spoke to her on her First Communion.

The third design is a full apron with a heart shaped bodice, two swan heads circling a couple, and a castle among leaves. The text reads "Love one another but make not a bond of love. Let it rather be a moving sea between the shores of your souls. Fill each other's cup but drink not from one cup. Give your hearts, but not into each others keeping. For only the hand of life can contain your hearts...For what knowest thou, O woman, whether thou shalt save thy husband. Or how knowest thou, O man, whether thou shalt save thy wife. As the Lord hath called every one, so let him walk." This design is based upon Christine's short marriage from age 18-22, the idealism, and the reality. The couple is from her wedding photo.

The fourth apron depicts a baby amidst plants growing in Dixie cups. The text reads "I told the doctor that I thought I was pregnant. We'll see, he said, and handed me a Dixie cup to pee in. I figured that this must be like Kindergarten when the teacher gave me a seed. I planted it in a Dixie cup to watch it grow." This design is about Christine's first pregnancy at the age of 21, again full of idealism. Her daughter, Amber, was born at home with a midwife.

A fifth more recent design by Ms. Ilewski also includes an apron. *On the Edge II* uses the actual apron collaged into the piece as the woman's dress. The bibbed portion cloaks the woman's upper torso. The apron ties over the shoulders and around the lower body act like 'wings' or perhaps tree limbs, both binding and freeing. It is acrylic on fabric and measures 48 by 52 inches.

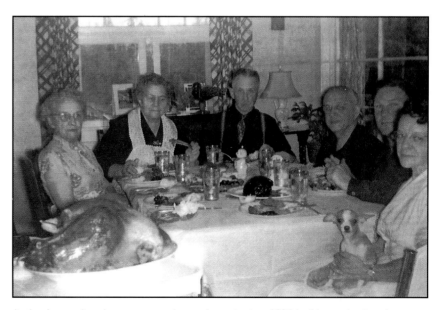

Author's grandmother, aunts, uncles, and cousins in a 1936 holiday gathering. Aunt Nelle is wearing her *good* apron with the rickrack edging.

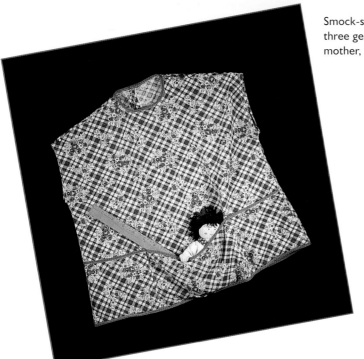

Smock-style child's cotton apron with a back button closure and three generous pockets, circa 1950, made by the author's mother, Eilene Paulson, for the author and her sister.

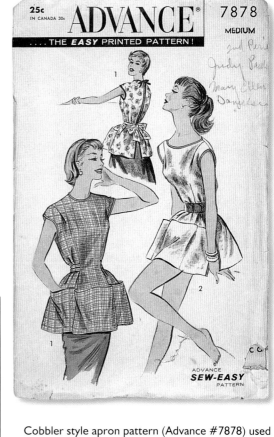

Cobbler style apron pattern (Advance #7878) used by the author in her high school freshman home economics class (1959-60). Her name and the name of the girl with whom she shared the pattern are penciled on the front.

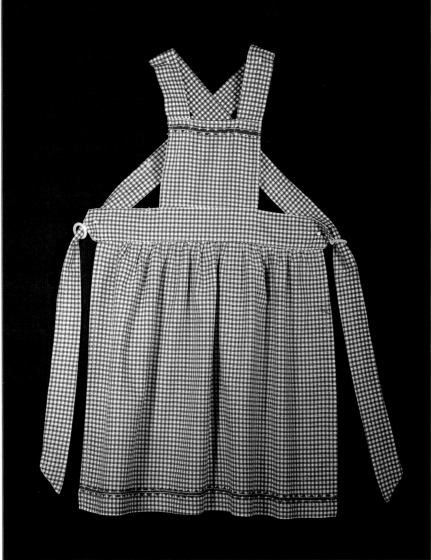

Pinafore-style child's cotton apron with bib, shoulder straps, and red rickrack, circa 1950, made by the author's mother, Eilene Paulson, for the author and her sister.

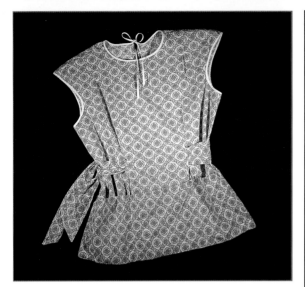

Cobbler apron made by the author during her freshman home economics class; from the collection of the author.

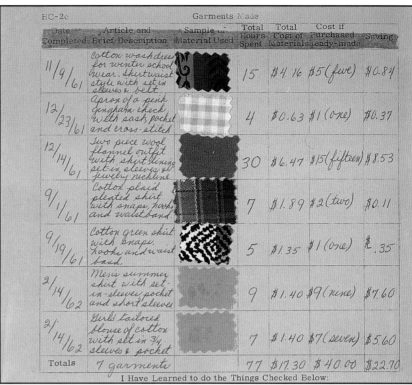

HC-2c	Garments Made					
Date Completed	Article and Brief Description	Sample of Material Used	Total Hours Spent	Total Cost of Materials	Cost if Purchased ready-made	Saving
11/9/61	Cotton wash dress for winter school wear. Shirtwaist style with set in sleeves & belt		15	$4.16	$5 (five)	$0.84
12/23/61	Apron of a pink gingham check with sash pocket and cross-stitch		4	$0.63	$1 (one)	$0.37
12/14/61	Two piece wool flannel outfit with skirt lining set-in sleeves & jewelry neckline		30	$6.47	$15 (fifteen)	$8.53
9/1/61	Cotton plaid pleated skirt with snaps, hook and waistband		7	$1.89	$2 (two)	$0.11
9/19/61	Cotton green skirt with snaps, hooks and waist band		5	$1.35	$1 (one)	$.35
2/14/62	Men's summer shirt with set-in sleeves pocket and short sleeves		9	$1.40	$9 (nine)	$7.60
2/14/62	Girls tailored blouse of cotton with set in 3/4 sleeves & pocket		7	$1.40	$7 (seven)	$5.60
Totals	7 garments		77	$17.30	$40.00	$22.70

I Have Learned to do the Things Checked Below:

Sample swatch and details about the gingham apron made by the author for her grandmother, from the author's 1961 4-H record book.

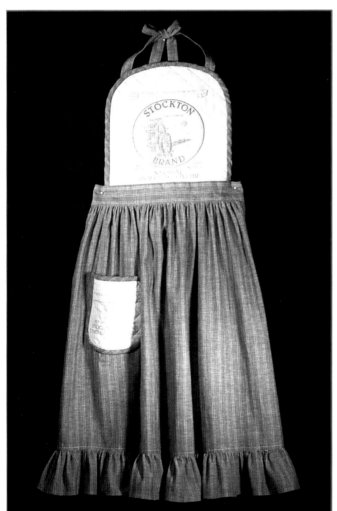

Apron made from a recycled cotton *Stockton Roller Mill* flour sack, quilting by the author, circa 1990; from the collection of the author.

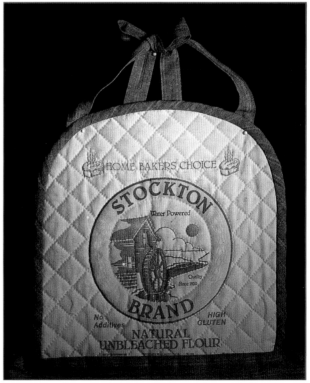

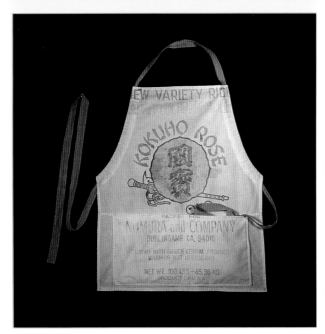

Apron made from a recycled cotton *Kokuho Rose* rice sack, sadly faded from intensive use and repeated launderings, circa 1990; from the collection of the author.

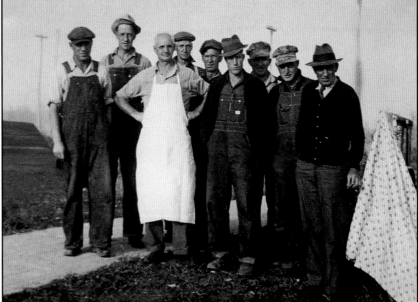

The cook stands out prominently, bare-headed, hands on his hips, proudly sporting an extra long white bibbed apron.

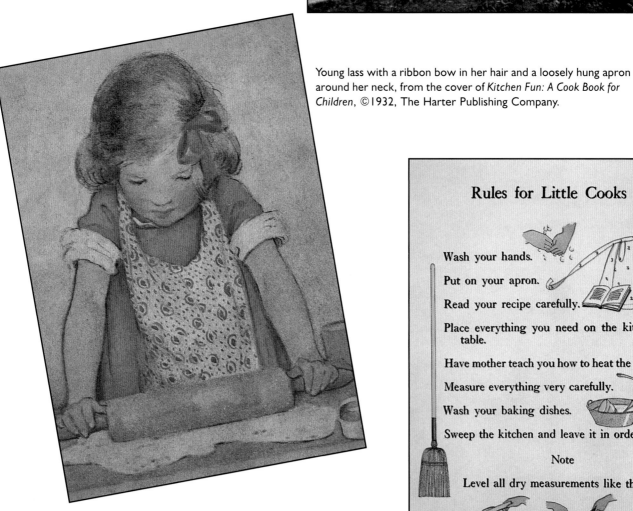

Young lass with a ribbon bow in her hair and a loosely hung apron around her neck, from the cover of *Kitchen Fun: A Cook Book for Children*, ©1932, The Harter Publishing Company.

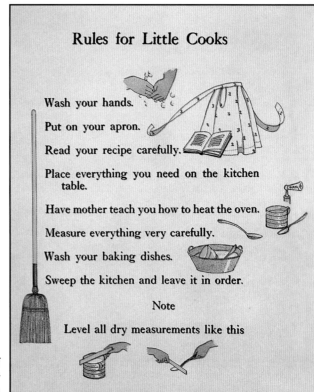

Rules for Little Cooks

Wash your hands.

Put on your apron.

Read your recipe carefully.

Place everything you need on the kitchen table.

Have mother teach you how to heat the oven.

Measure everything very carefully.

Wash your baking dishes.

Sweep the kitchen and leave it in order.

Note

Level all dry measurements like this

"Rules for Little Cooks," from the inside front cover of *Kitchen Fun: A Cook Book for Children*, ©1932, The Harter Publishing Company.

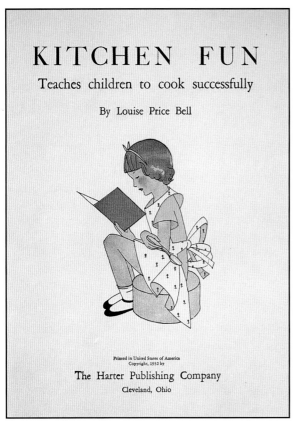

Little girl in widely flared pinafore style apron with long sashes and large bow, *Kitchen Fun: A Cook Book for Children*, page 1, ©1932, The Harter Publishing Company.

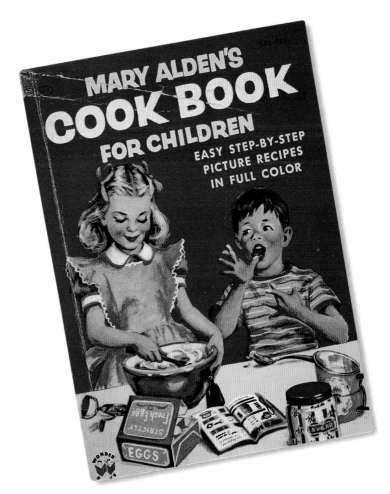

Girl in a ruffled and sashed gray apron, from the cover of *Mary Alden's Cookbook for Children*, © 1955, Wonder Books, Inc.

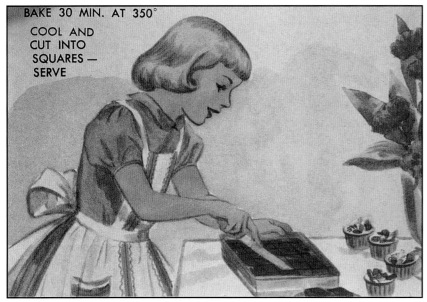

Girl in a white bibbed apron with colorful trim down the front and across the patch pocket, *Mary Alden's Cookbook for Children*, page 37, ©1955, Wonder Books, Inc.

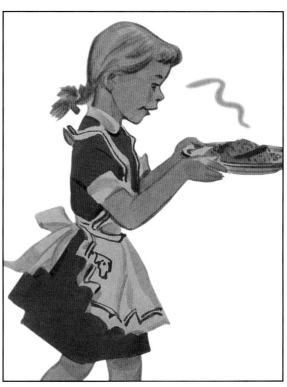

Pig-tailed girl outfitted in a stylish white pinafore apron with red decoration, *Mary Alden's Cookbook for Children*, page 49, ©1955, Wonder Books, Inc.

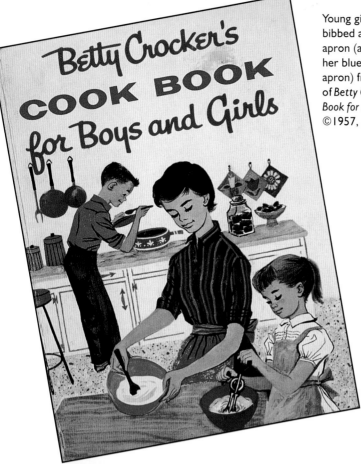

Young girl in a pink bibbed and sashed apron (and Mother in her blue gathered half apron) from the cover of *Betty Crocker's Cook Book for Boys and Girls*, ©1957, Golden Press.

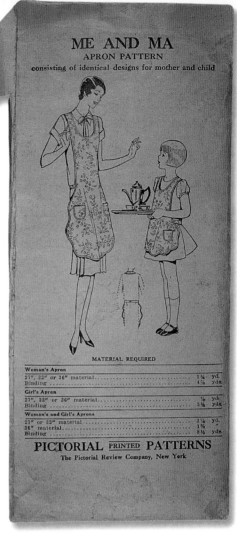

"Me and Ma" apron pattern consisting of identical designs for mother and child, ©1925, The Pictorial Review Company.

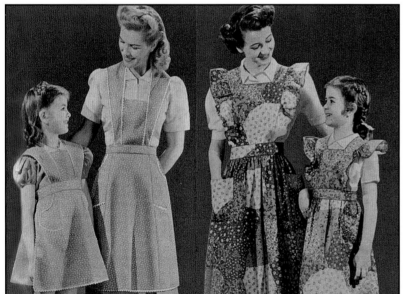

Mothers and daughters in look alike bibbed and pinafored aprons, from the 1942-43 Fall/Winter Montgomery Ward Catalog, ©Montgomery Ward.

Mother in her half apron and a child in her coverall apron, from page 31 of *The Elson Pupil's Hand Chart*.

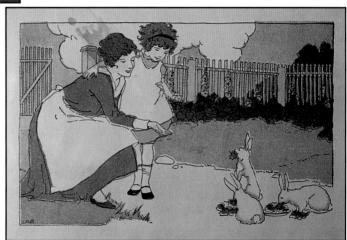

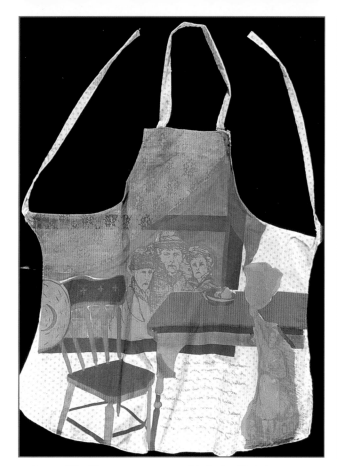

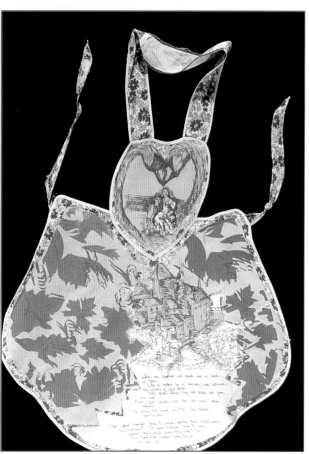

Apron #3, screen print on cotton fabric, by Christine Ilewski. *Photo courtesy of Christine Ilewski.*

Apron #1, silk screen on cotton fabric, by Christine Ilewski. *Photo courtesy of Christine Ilewski.*

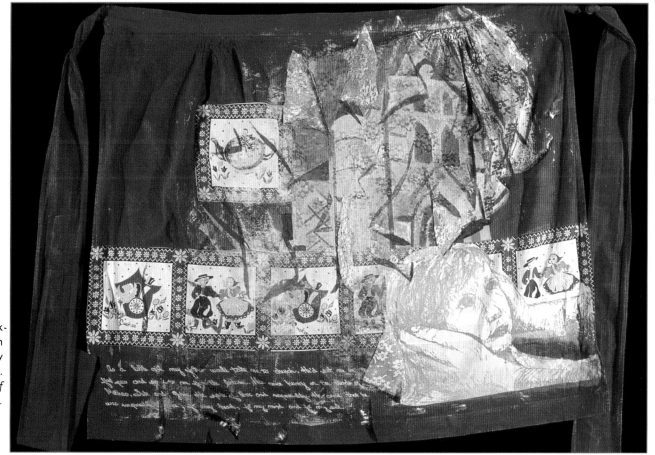

Apron #2, silk-screen print on cotton fabric, by Christine Ilewski. *Photo courtesy of Christine Ilewski.*

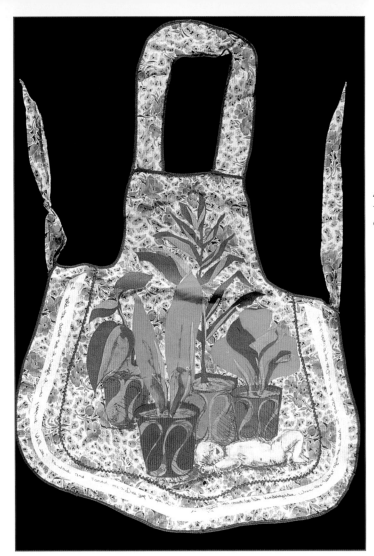

Apron #4, screen print on cotton fabric, by Christine Ilewski. *Photo courtesy of Christine Ilewski.*

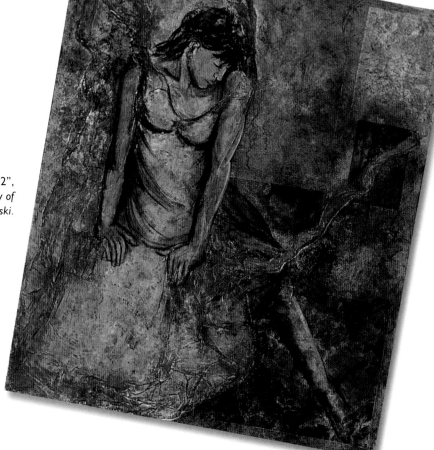

Apron #5, acrylic on fabric, 48" x 52", by Christine Ilewski. *Photo courtesy of Christine Ilewski.*

Section One

FABRIC STYLES

Every Color Under the Sun: Gingham Aprons

One of the most popular apron styles of the mid-twentieth century was the cross stitched gingham apron. Almost everybody can recall this 'checkered' kitchen staple. If you hadn't actually made or worn one yourself, you probably had a mother or grandmother that did. Many people think of the two—apron and gingham—as synonymous.

The word gingham is a derivative of the Malay *gingan* or *genggang*, meaning checkered cloth. It is a woven yarn-dyed (as opposed to printed) cotton in plain weave. It is usually in stripes or checks, of two or more colors, and used for dresses, aprons, etc. Gingham varies in the width of the check from extremely narrow (one-sixteenth of an inch) to very wide (one inch). The most common widths are one-eighth and one-fourth inch.

Gingham cloth was available for 18¢ a yard in the 1935-36 Sears Catalog. Billed as "Smart Ginghams for a Gay Life and a Long Life," they were "boilfast and of a fine beautiful weave." Additional descriptions read:

> You can picture how stunning this new gingham is; but we wish you could actually see and feel it! It's so smooth. . . so fine and even! Tailors perfectly; pleats crisply. Use it for dresses and gay little suits; for curtains.

Propelled into the modern age of synthetic fibers and blended fabrics 35 years later, the 1971 Fall/Winter Montgomery Wards Catalog offered "woven checks in two qualities." The first is a blend, described as:

> No ironing needed, 65% Dupont Dacron® polyester, 35% cotton, "spot-check" eases out stains, available in nine colors—red, turquoise, yellow, lilac, blue, pink, black, orange, and lime. (The featured model opted for lime.)

A more economical option was the 100% yarn-dyed cotton, machine washable (hot), little or no ironing gingham at 67¢ per yard.

The range of available colors was like the rainbow. Neutral colors in beige, brown, and black were also available. The most preferred colors seem to be red, pink, turquoise, and blue. Red and blue, of course, are universally favored colors. Perhaps pink was selected for its traditional "feminine" connotation. Turquoise was simply a fashionable color in the 1950s and 1960s.

Cross stitching seemed to go hand-in-hand with gingham aprons. The evenly spaced checks provide a naturally gridded background for the placement of stitches and designs. If one could count, and if one could thread a needle and take a simple stitch, the world of cross stitched

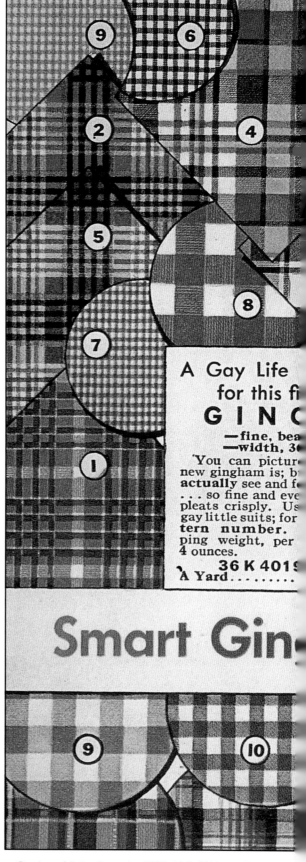

Gingham fabrics from the 1935-36 Fall/Winter Sears Catalog, page 398, described as "Smart Ginghams— A Gay Life, A Long Life, for this Fine Brilliant Gingham, 18¢ a yard."

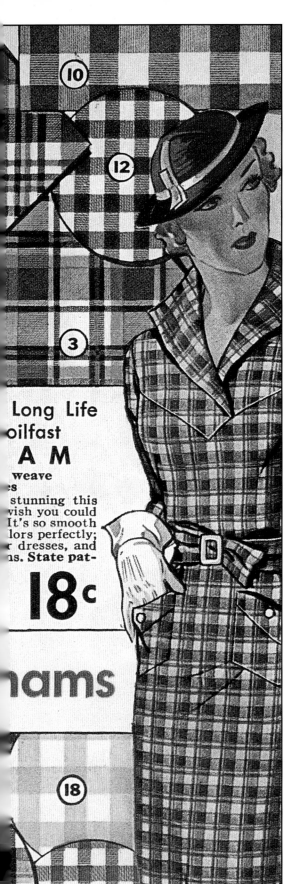

gingham aprons was open. No knowledge of complicated embroidery stitches was required. A basic in-and-out stitch was all that was needed. And a generous dose of perseverance.

Many makers of gingham aprons did not end with the cross stitched design. Other embellishments included rickrack, smocking, pulled thread, and appliquéd ornaments. Each added individual elegance to the apron. Finely executed cross stitches combined with carefully placed ornaments usually made a pleasing design and added the "finishing touch."

Fifteen examples of gingham aprons are pictured. They have the following parameters: All are one-eighth inch gingham, all have cross stitching, and all have two sashes and one patch pocket. Their distinctiveness lies in their colors (fifteen delicious hues) and their cross stitch designs (fifteen impressive patterns). They are nearly equally divided between pleated (no waistband) and gathered (with waistband) styles.

All fifteen aprons have been photographed in a similar horizontal format with one sash draped at the side, the other sash opened and arranged across the top. This makes it convenient to compare details such as the size of the apron, length and width of sashes, shape of sash ends, waistband style, and pockets. Each apron also has a detailed close-up photo of the cross stitched designs.

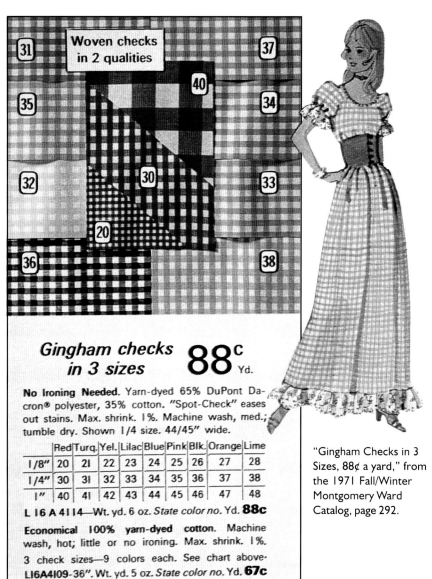

Woven checks in 2 qualities

Gingham checks in 3 sizes 88c Yd.

No Ironing Needed. Yarn-dyed 65% DuPont Dacron® polyester, 35% cotton. "Spot-Check" eases out stains. Max. shrink. 1%. Machine wash, med.; tumble dry. Shown 1/4 size. 44/45" wide.

	Red	Turq.	Yel.	Lilac	Blue	Pink	Blk.	Orange	Lime
1/8"	20	21	22	23	24	25	26	27	28
1/4"	30	31	32	33	34	35	36	37	38
1"	40	41	42	43	44	45	46	47	48

L 16 A 4114—Wt. yd. 6 oz. *State color no.* Yd. **88c**

Economical 100% yarn-dyed cotton. Machine wash, hot; little or no ironing. Max. shrink. 1%. 3 check sizes—9 colors each. See chart above. L16A4109-36". Wt. yd. 5 oz. *State color no.* Yd. **67c**

"Gingham Checks in 3 Sizes, 88¢ a yard," from the 1971 Fall/Winter Montgomery Ward Catalog, page 292.

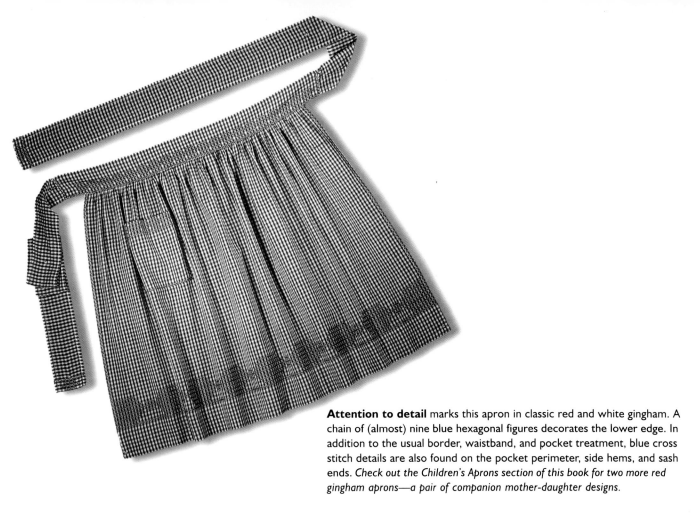

Attention to detail marks this apron in classic red and white gingham. A chain of (almost) nine blue hexagonal figures decorates the lower edge. In addition to the usual border, waistband, and pocket treatment, blue cross stitch details are also found on the pocket perimeter, side hems, and sash ends. *Check out the Children's Aprons section of this book for two more red gingham aprons—a pair of companion mother-daughter designs.*

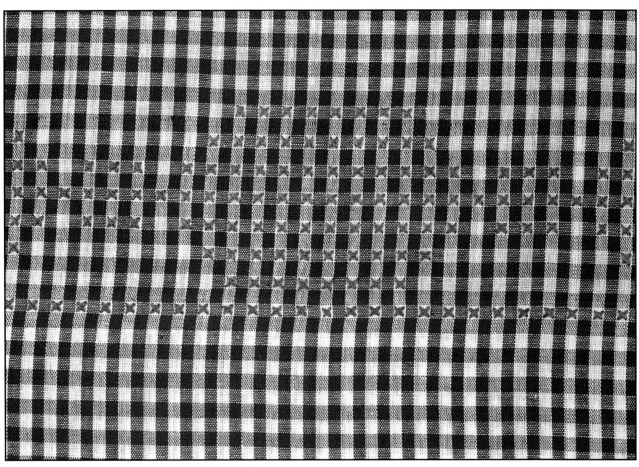

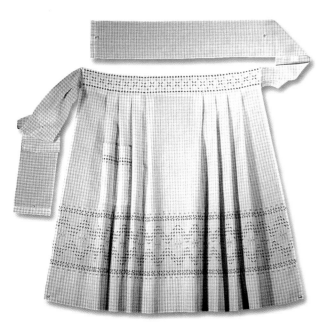

How did this apron ever come to be? Doesn't it just fly in the face of what your mother said about pink and red not going together? Nonetheless, here is a six-inch border of horizontal lines, zigzags, and hexagonal stars in **crossed and uncrossed stitches** of pink and red.

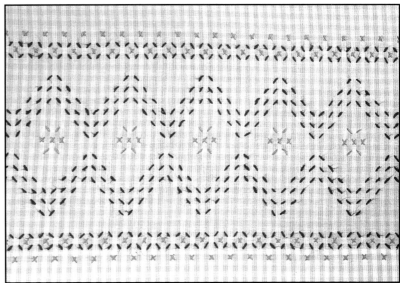

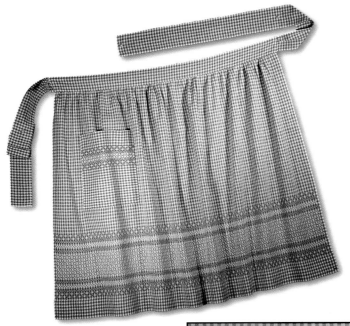

The flavor of orange sherbet is evident in this gathered gingham apron. Large X's stitched in white embroidery thread and smaller X's in orange and white carefully placed in single rows make an effective six inch border. An abbreviated design is also stitched across the pocket. This is a fine example of the creation of lightness (in the center of the border) by placing white cross stitches over the dark (orange) squares, and creation of darkness (top and bottom of the border) by placing dark (orange) cross stitches over the white spaces.

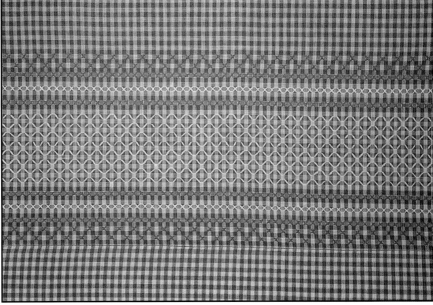

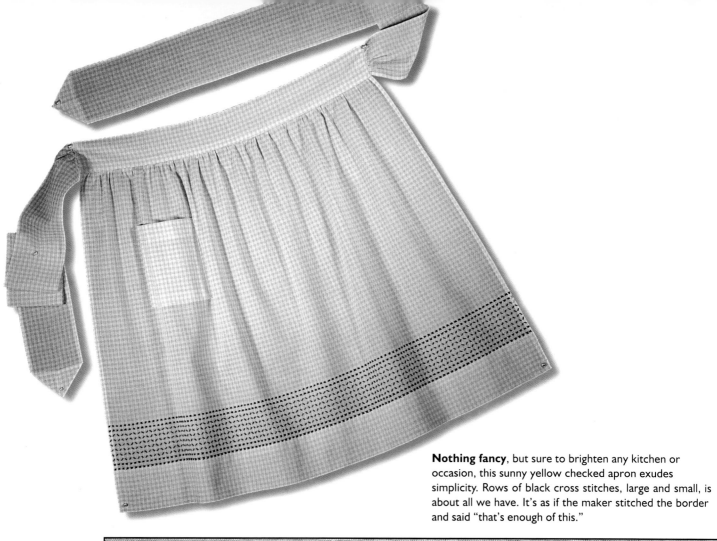

Nothing fancy, but sure to brighten any kitchen or occasion, this sunny yellow checked apron exudes simplicity. Rows of black cross stitches, large and small, is about all we have. It's as if the maker stitched the border and said "that's enough of this."

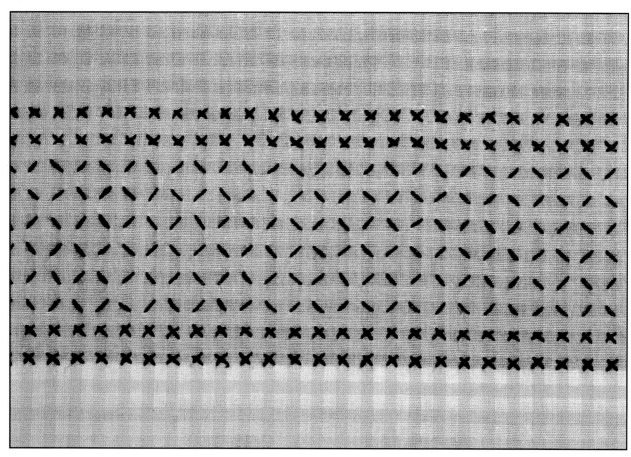

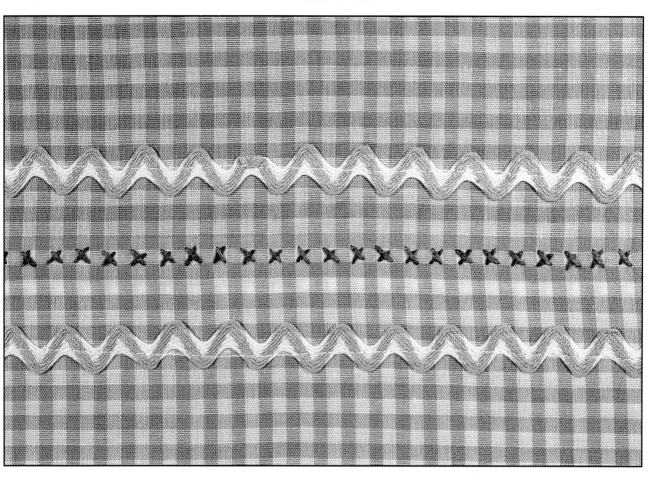

Cross stitch and rickrack go hand-in-hand on this pistachio-green pleated design. The pocket and skirt are outlined with a solitary row of tiny green X's. Dual color rickrack is machine-stitched on the pocket, waistline, and lower edge. Although this is the only example in this section, rickrack was frequently combined with cross stitching on gingham aprons of the 1950s and 1960s.

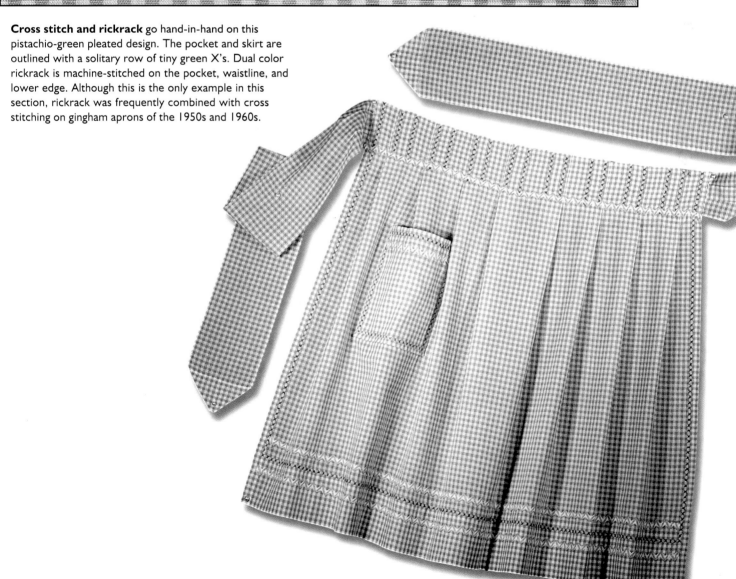

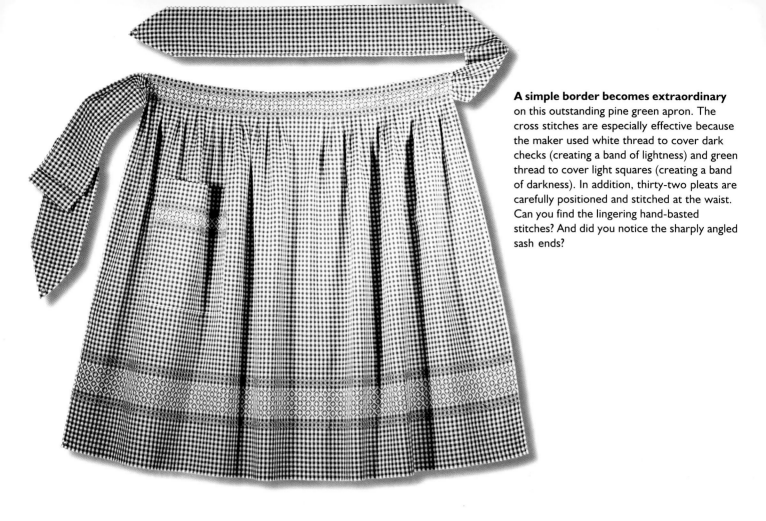

A simple border becomes extraordinary on this outstanding pine green apron. The cross stitches are especially effective because the maker used white thread to cover dark checks (creating a band of lightness) and green thread to cover light squares (creating a band of darkness). In addition, thirty-two pleats are carefully positioned and stitched at the waist. Can you find the lingering hand-basted stitches? And did you notice the sharply angled sash ends?

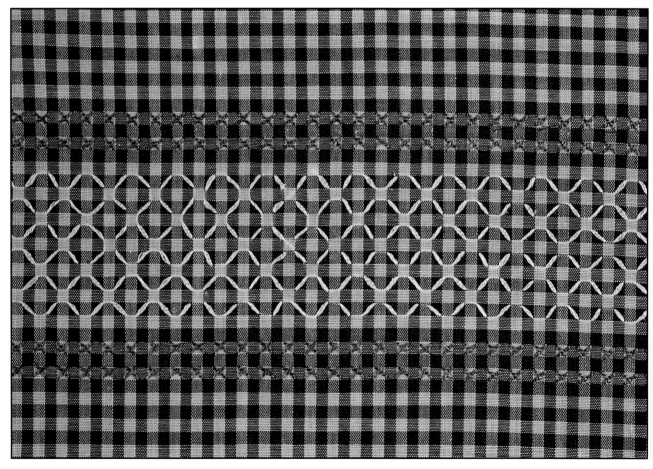

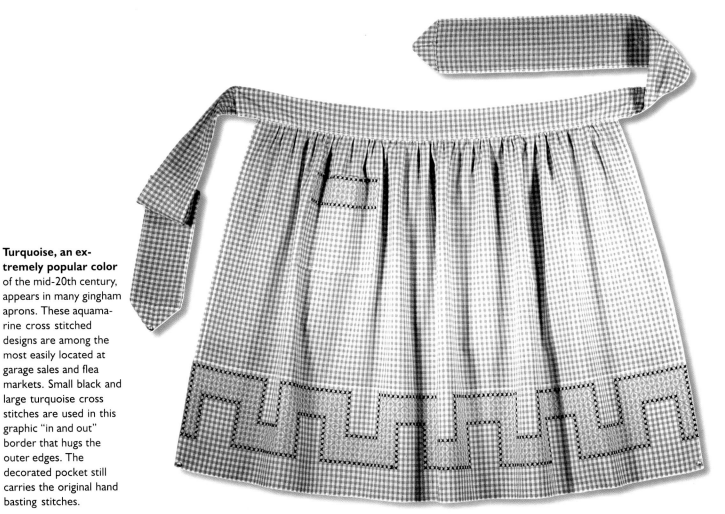

Turquoise, an extremely popular color of the mid-20th century, appears in many gingham aprons. These aquamarine cross stitched designs are among the most easily located at garage sales and flea markets. Small black and large turquoise cross stitches are used in this graphic "in and out" border that hugs the outer edges. The decorated pocket still carries the original hand basting stitches.

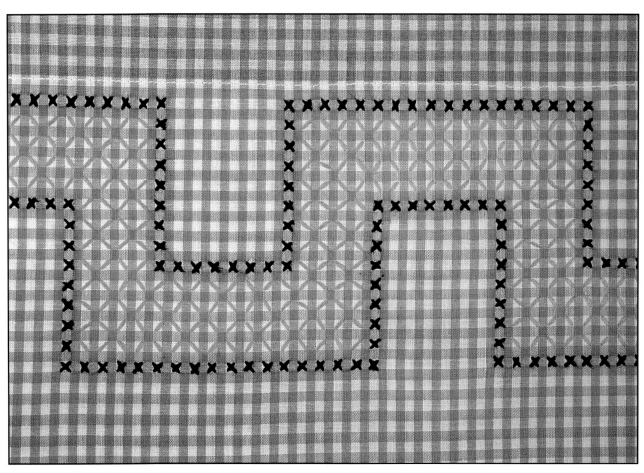

Double stranded white embroidery thread is used in the lined and flowered border of this **easy-on-the-eyes** sky blue gathered apron. A double row of miniature X's also appears on the banded pocket. The extra wide waist-band is accented with a triple row of stitches with interspersed spaces.

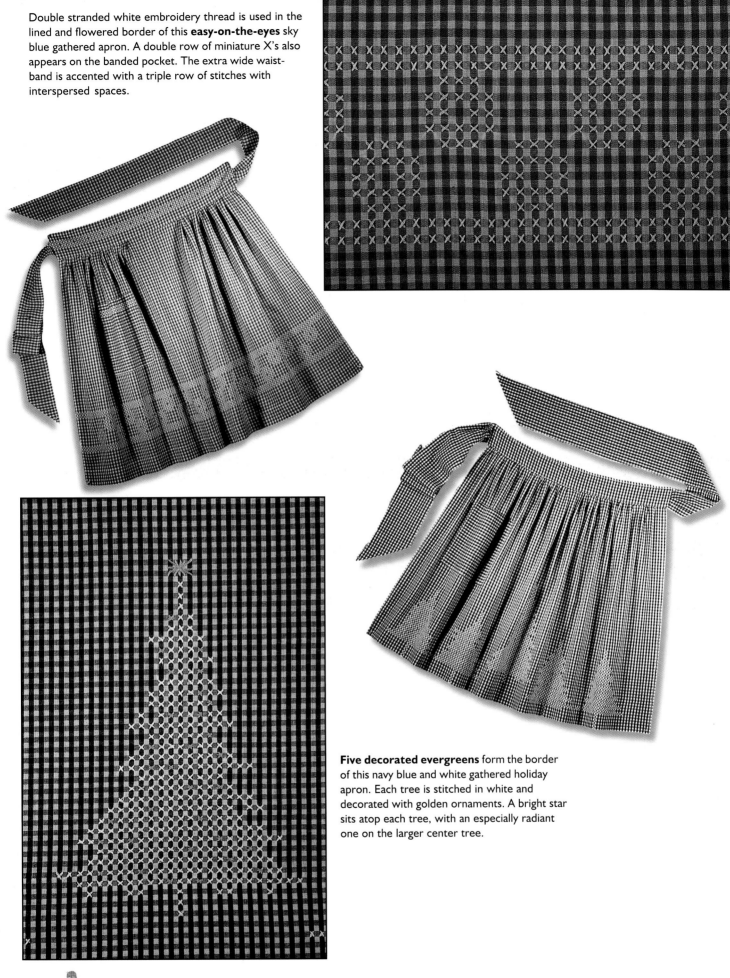

Five decorated evergreens form the border of this navy blue and white gathered holiday apron. Each tree is stitched in white and decorated with golden ornaments. A bright star sits atop each tree, with an especially radiant one on the larger center tree.

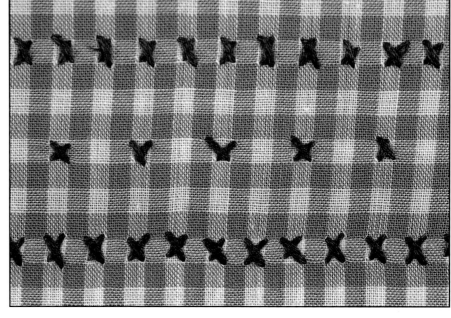

Some called it lavender, others orchid or lilac. No matter what label was applied it was a popular color of the 1950s and 1960s, as evidenced in this **monochromatic design**. A narrow border of single and double spaced X's traverses the lower edge, and the pocket and sides are similarly decorated. *Look for another lavender gingham apron on page 138 in The Color Purple section. It has wide one-inch checks and rickrack trim.*

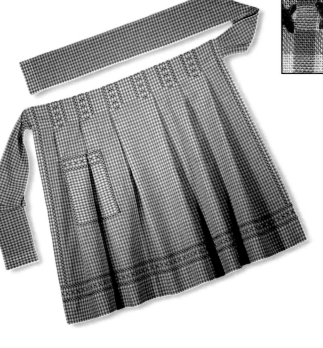

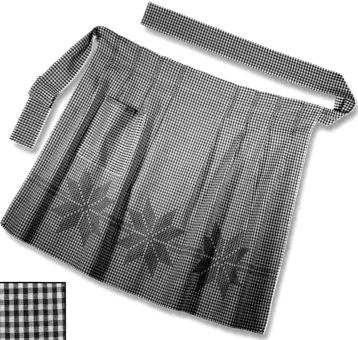

Three **huge cross stitched stars** dominate the border of this purple and white gingham apron. Each star is composed of eight parallelograms and measures about seven inches from point to point. A row of diagonal stitches trails between the stars. Larger X's highlight the waistband and pocket. *Everything* on this apron is hand sewn—cross stitches, lower hem, side hems, pleats, waistband attachment, sash hems and ends, pocket appliqué, *everything*.

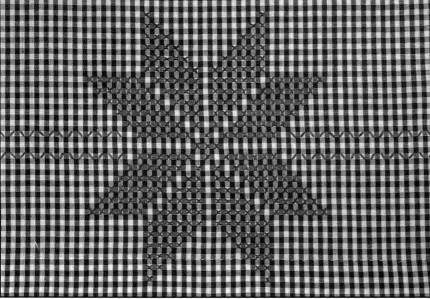

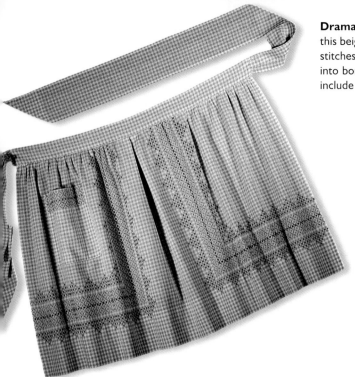

Dramatic cornered designs are the center of attention in this beige gathered gingham apron. Chocolate brown cross stitches in two sizes (1/8 and 3/8 inches) drop from the waist into border style designs with triangular edges. Added details include a center box pleat and pocket decoration.

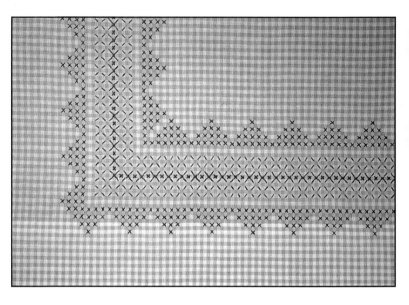

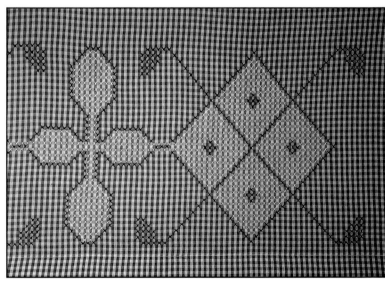

A graphic tripartite design of sizable squares set on point and a lantern shaped motif dominate this cinnamon brown apron. Dense cross stitching with creamy colored embroidery thread creates a feeling of lightness on the shapes in this **black, brown, and beige** design.

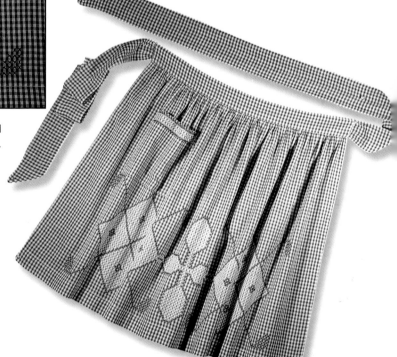

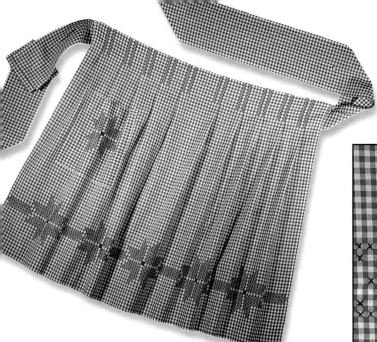

Did you even know that gingham check was **available in gray**? Probably not very common, but here's evidence that it was not only available, but used in aprons, as well. When combined with cherry red embroidery thread in this lovely eight-point star border, the effect is quite dramatic. Precise pleats and vertical cross stitches highlight the waistline. What about the centers of the stars? They are miniature *Teneriffe* lace designs, each barely 3/8 of an inch square.

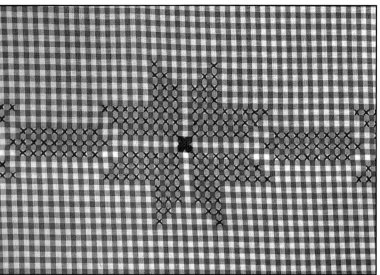

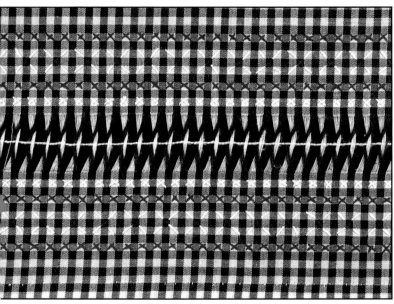

Tiny red and large white cross stitches combine with a one-inch line of **pulled thread work** on this black gingham checked fabric. Horizontal threads have been removed and the remaining vertical stitches have been grouped and interwoven with white embroidery floss. Additional stitches accent the pocket and pleated waistline, and also the ends of the sashes!

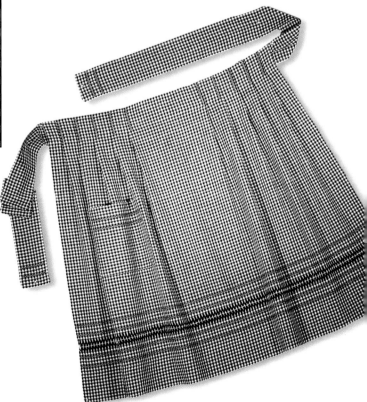

Floral Arrangements

We really need only one word to describe the aprons in this section—beautiful. During the planning stages of this book, a chapter was tentatively designated "Showcase: Extraordinary Aprons and All-time Favorites." As it turned out most of the aprons that made their way into that section were floral designs, often large showy patterns of sumptuous colors. Eventually the section was fine tuned and became *only* aprons of floral design.

The aprons included here are strewn with roses, pansies, rose buds, morning glories, carnations, and more roses. They are covered with bouquets, sprays, garlands, borders full of flowers, and vases full of flowers. Even pockets full of flowers. The blooms and blossoms appear in fine prints and bold images, rickracked and hand painted. They are all quite breathtaking. Descriptions just don't do them justice.

Fourteen of those floral arrangements were selected for your viewing pleasure. Go ahead and feast your eyes on them—just because they're beautiful!

That's not all...there are additional floral design aprons scattered throughout the book. Watch for the anthurium, orchids, tulips, and various unidentifiable stylized flowers.

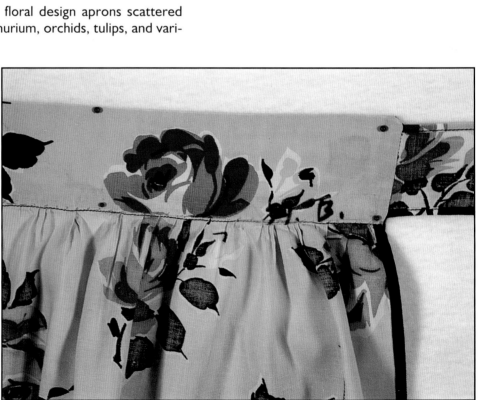

Giant red roses and dainty yellow rosebuds on a mint green background add up to **an undisputed American beauty**. The gently scalloped lower edge is trimmed and edged with black bias. A deep pocket has a mock flap and black trim. The initials "A. B." have been inscribed with blue marker on the inside waistband, as if to lay claim. If this were my apron, I'd want it back, too.

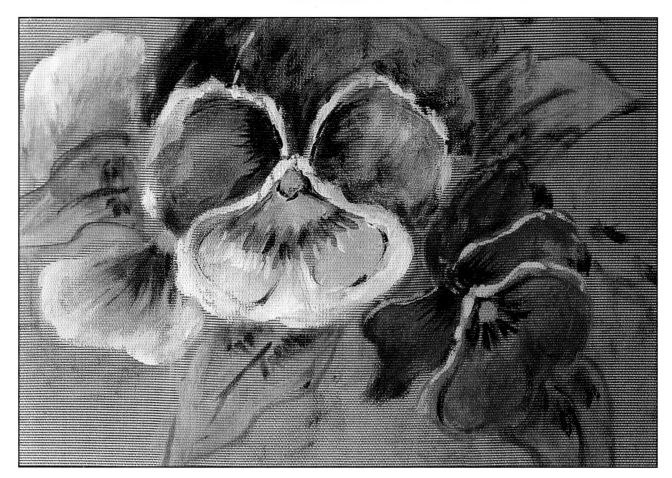

Luxurious shiny pale peach taffeta serves as the background for these gorgeous hand-painted pansies. The rainbow of colors in **emerging buds and full blooms** is also highlighted on the roomy waistband and the uniquely shaped hexagonal pocket. Sash ends are also embellished with hand-painted purple pansies.

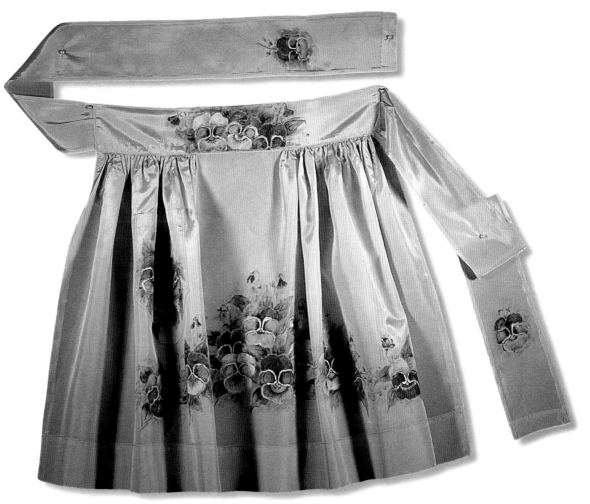

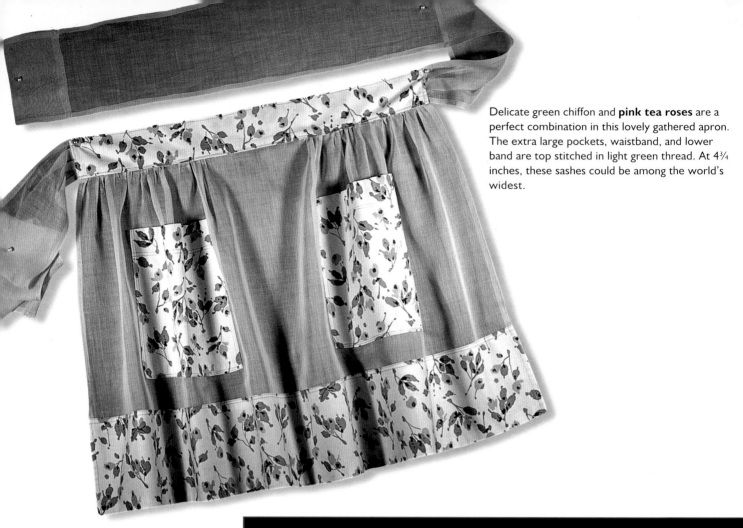

Delicate green chiffon and **pink tea roses** are a perfect combination in this lovely gathered apron. The extra large pockets, waistband, and lower band are top stitched in light green thread. At 4¾ inches, these sashes could be among the world's widest.

You could gather **a bouquet of red roses** from this pleated organdy and percale apron. As if roses weren't enough, additional enhancements include a gently curved lower edge, white rickrack edging, and an Empire waistline. The twin pockets are also edged with rickrack.

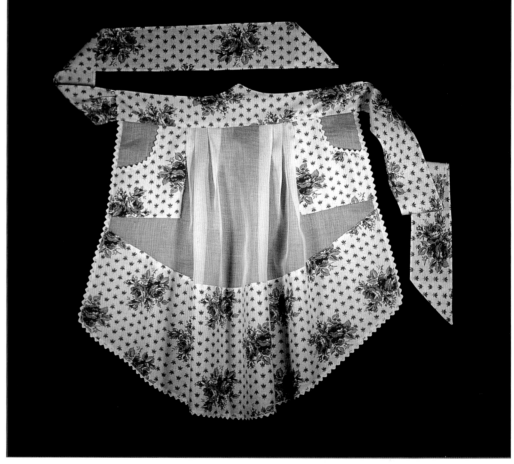

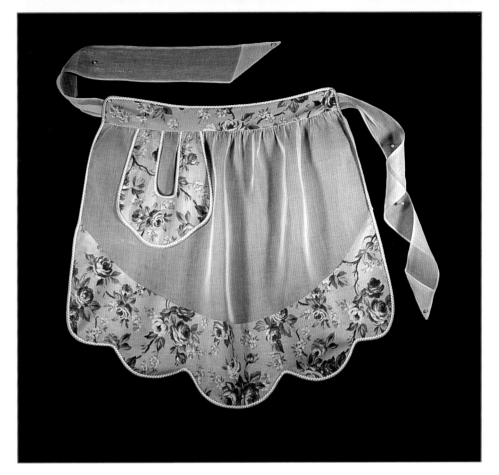

An unusually shaped **front entry pocket** is the focal point of this sky blue gathered apron of organdy and cotton percale. Miniature white rickrack outlines the waistband, pocket edge and opening, and lower edge. The curved organdy, gently scalloped lower edge, and rounded pocket result in an especially satisfying design.

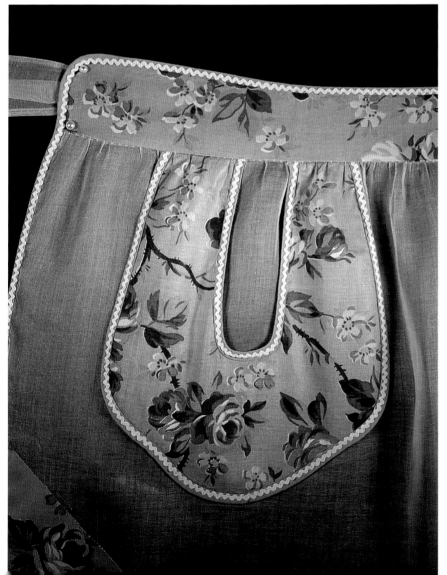

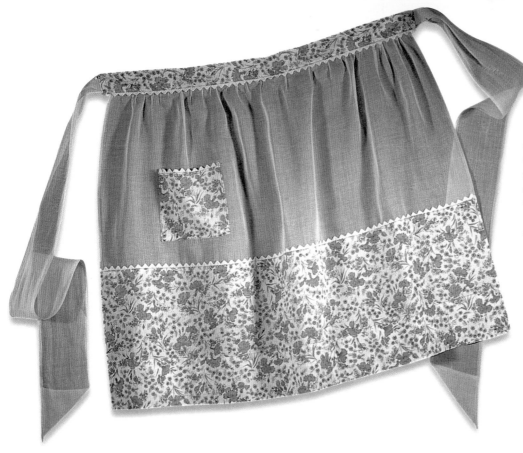

A floral print in **turquoise and peach** is complemented with lightweight pale aqua organdy in this easy-to-construct apron. White rickrack accents the waistband, lower band, and square pocket. The sashes are deeply pleated and the waistline lightly gathered.

An overskirt of baby blue organdy lends **a sense of mystery** to this flared apron. Floral sprays of blue and pink flowers on pure white cotton and white rickrack edging convey a clean airy feeling. The contour appliquéd pockets give a triple-layer illusion.

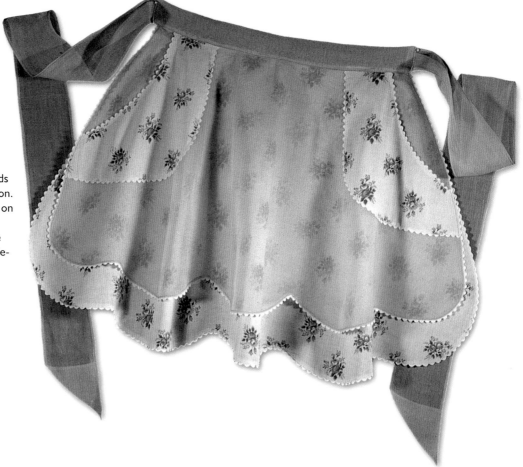

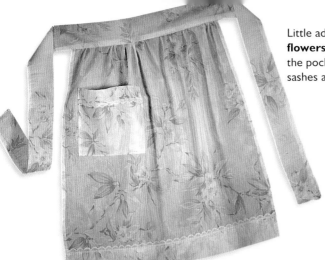

Little adornment is needed on these **showy and suggestive flowers** of translucent nylon. Pale pink scalloped edging on the pocket and hem lends to the subdued feeling. The sashes and waistband are simply constructed in one piece.

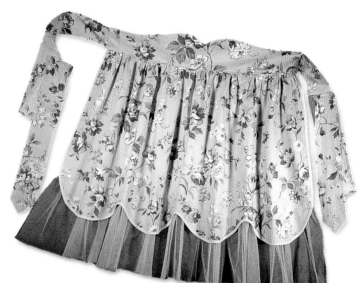

If favorites were selected, this might be among the lot. The beautiful display of flowers and foliage in **a rainbow of colors** is further enhanced with a doubled six-inch tulle ruffle. Yellow edging along the sides and scalloped lower edges adds just the right note of brightness. The "heart-shaped" waistband adds a classy final touch.

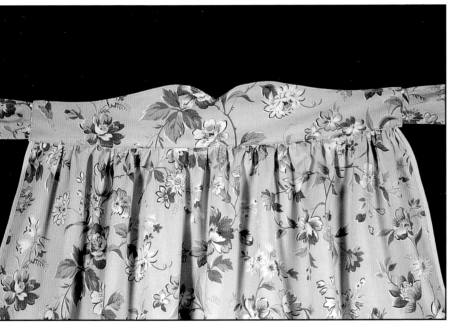

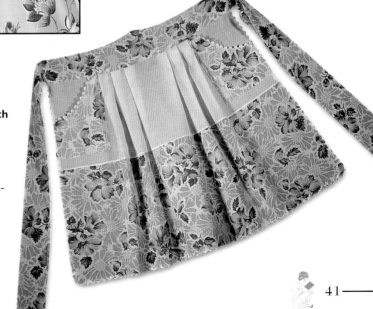

Here is proof that you can **say it with flowers**. The creator of this pleated apron relied on a rosy pink and sky blue floral print and white cotton lawn for a design of simple beauty. White rickrack is used for embellishment. A slightly shaped waistband completes the design.

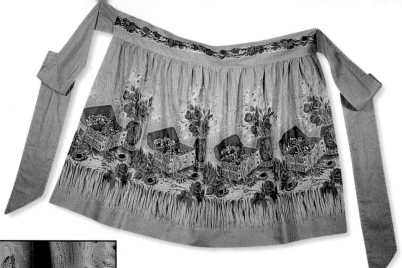

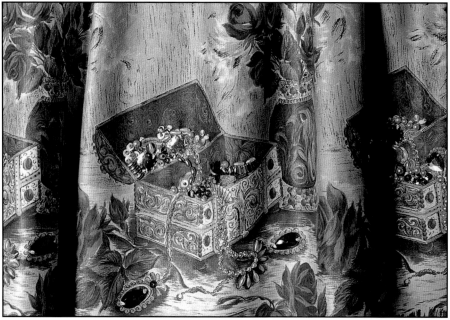

Perhaps the winner in the kitchen kitsch category, this **bejeweled and blue-rosed border print** apron is certain to catch the eye and carry the conversation. Treasure trunks overflow with beads, sequins, pearls, and sundry baubles. Who cares if there is no pocket?

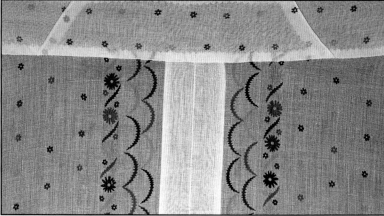

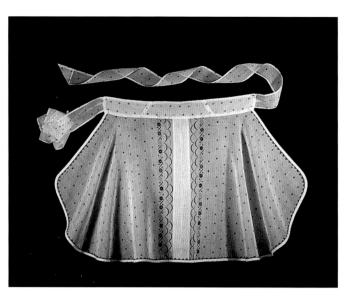

The center seam has become **a design element of its own** on this organdy apron. A border-printed floral design with the tiniest of flowers is cleverly centered, and red rickrack has been inserted and machine-zigzagged into the binding. Notice how the diagonal seams on the waistband enhance the center design.

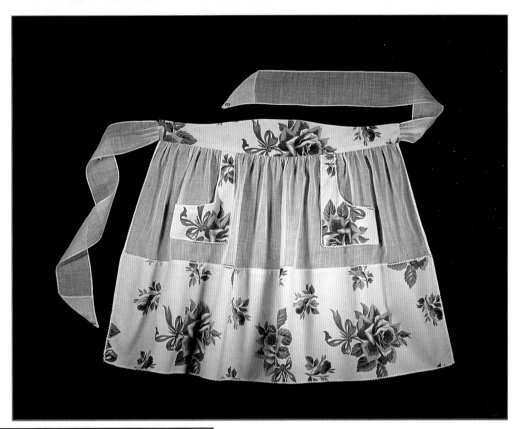

The soft pinks and corals of these showy roses are **certain to capture the attention** of guests. Buds and full blooms are embellished with blue ribbons and bows and greenery set against an eggshell background. Miniature white rickrack outlines the skirt and patch pockets, which are attached at the waist. Graceful curves top the waistband of this gathered organdy and cotton percale apron.

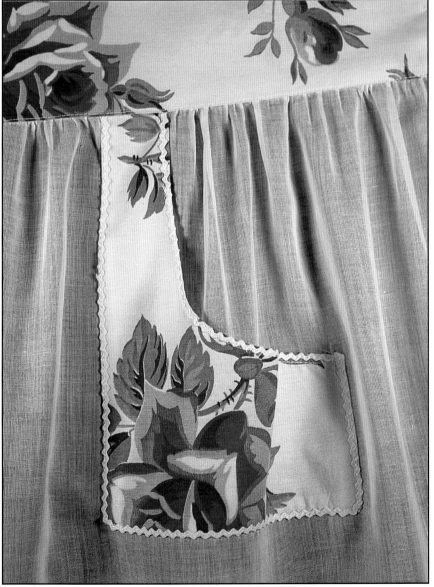

A Prevalence of Polka Dots

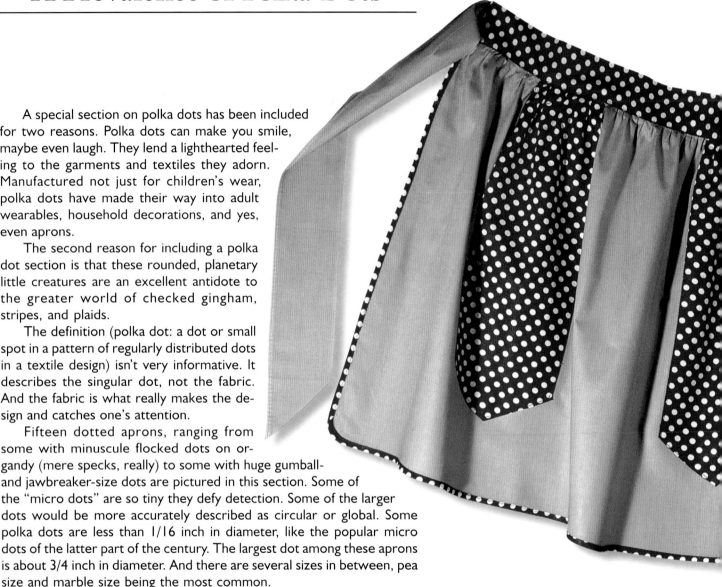

A special section on polka dots has been included for two reasons. Polka dots can make you smile, maybe even laugh. They lend a lighthearted feeling to the garments and textiles they adorn. Manufactured not just for children's wear, polka dots have made their way into adult wearables, household decorations, and yes, even aprons.

The second reason for including a polka dot section is that these rounded, planetary little creatures are an excellent antidote to the greater world of checked gingham, stripes, and plaids.

The definition (polka dot: a dot or small spot in a pattern of regularly distributed dots in a textile design) isn't very informative. It describes the singular dot, not the fabric. And the fabric is what really makes the design and catches one's attention.

Fifteen dotted aprons, ranging from some with minuscule flocked dots on organdy (mere specks, really) to some with huge gumball- and jawbreaker-size dots are pictured in this section. Some of the "micro dots" are so tiny they defy detection. Some of the larger dots would be more accurately described as circular or global. Some polka dots are less than 1/16 inch in diameter, like the popular micro dots of the latter part of the century. The largest dot among these aprons is about 3/4 inch in diameter. And there are several sizes in between, pea size and marble size being the most common.

The two customary polka dot arrangements are white spots against a colored background and colored spots against a white background. Of course, there are the inevitable variations, e.g., dots of mixed colors against white (some rather patriotic red, white, and blue examples are included), even mixed sizes against white. More often, however, the trend is toward consistent sizes, lending a uniformity and evenness to the fabric. Examples of all these arrangements are pictured.

An unusual white nylon organdy apron with red flocked dots is included. One of the few nylon aprons in the book, it is made from a wiry, non absorbent, not too practical fabric, a purely decorative design. It is a dotted organdy apron and I have coined a phrase to describe it—a "dot org" apron, borrowing from today's computer language.

Two examples of aprons with Swedish or huck weaving are also included. Using dotted organdy fabric, the threads of the embroidered design are literally connected dot-to-dot, the raised flocked dots serving as the grid work onto which the stitches are placed. (A third example of Swedish weaving is included in the *Needle Arts* section.)

Other things to look for in this section: 1. Dots that have been embellished with embroidery and transformed into flowers; 2. Dots that grace the prime examples of apron kitsch (his and her designs), evidence that the maker didn't regard the lowly polka dot very seriously; and 3. A breathtakingly beautiful pink polka-dotted and ruffled store-bought design.

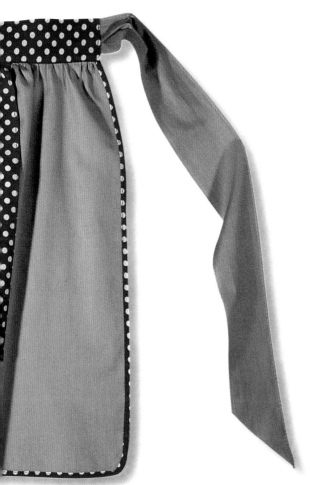

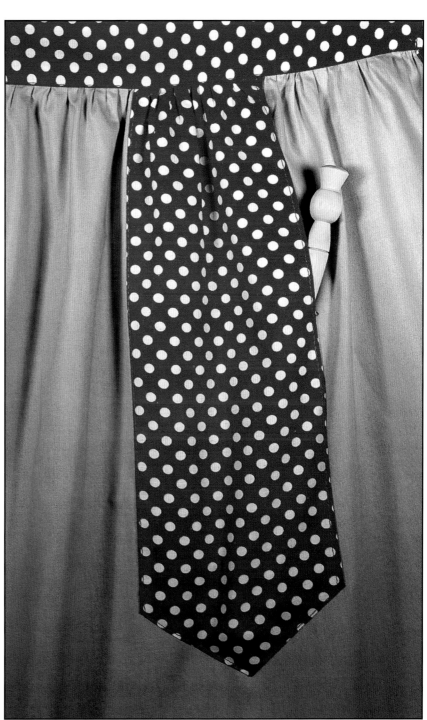

White pea-sized polka dots against a fire-engine red background are the eye-catchers in this classic **red, white, and sky blue** apron. The pointed and elongated panels double as deep pockets. The edges of this cotton gathered design are also trimmed with the polka dot fabric. Not so obvious are the hidden side entries to the pockets.

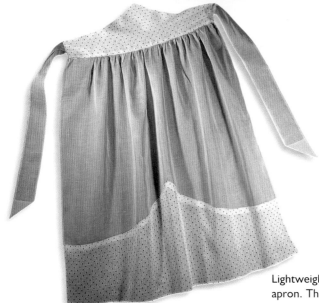

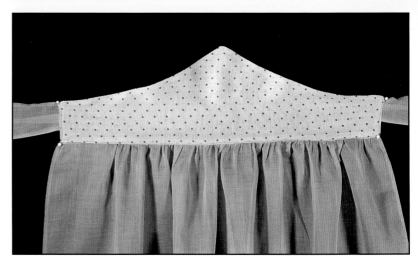

Lightweight cotton dotted and solid organdy in **shades of blue** is the mainstay of this dressy apron. The skirt is gathered and the oh-so-short sashes are pleated. Gently raised lines (Empire) at the waistband and the lower edge complete this delicate see-through design.

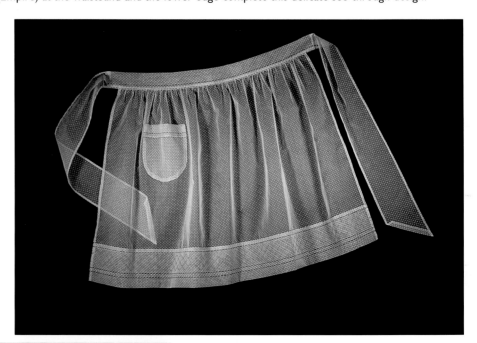

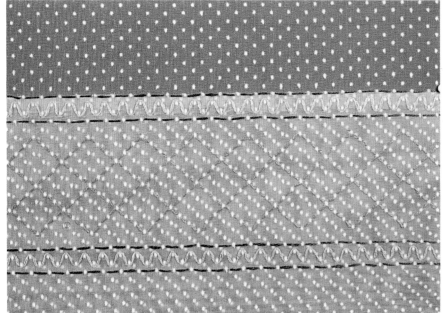

Dotted nylon organdy (sometimes called dotted Swiss) was a popular fabric in the 1950s and 1960s. Permanently flocked white dots served as the grid work for huck style embroidery. Two **shades of green** embroidery thread are worked into the border of this light green organdy apron. The modest diamond and zigzag pattern is repeated, in part, on the U-shaped pocket and waistband. *Additional examples of Swedish 'huck' embroidery are located in the Needle Arts and Pretty in Pink sections.*

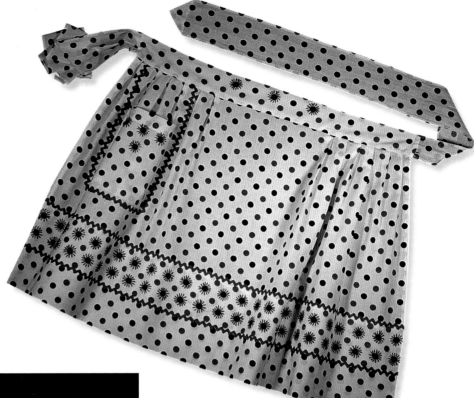

More than mere polka dots, this design includes rickrack and lazy daisy embroidery stitches. Blue dots are transformed into flowerets, and red rickrack creates borders around the pocket and along the lower edge of this pleated apron. The rickrack is attached by hand, with red embroidery floss. Notice the flower accents on the pocket and waistband.

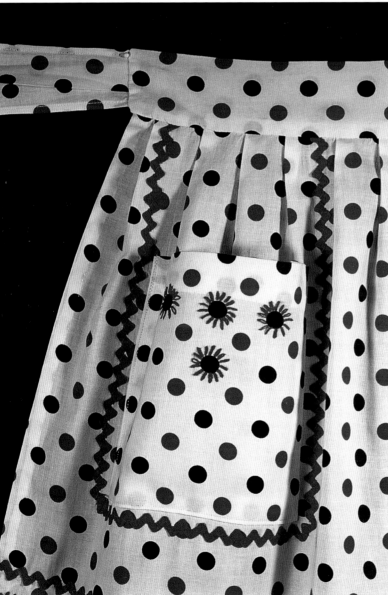

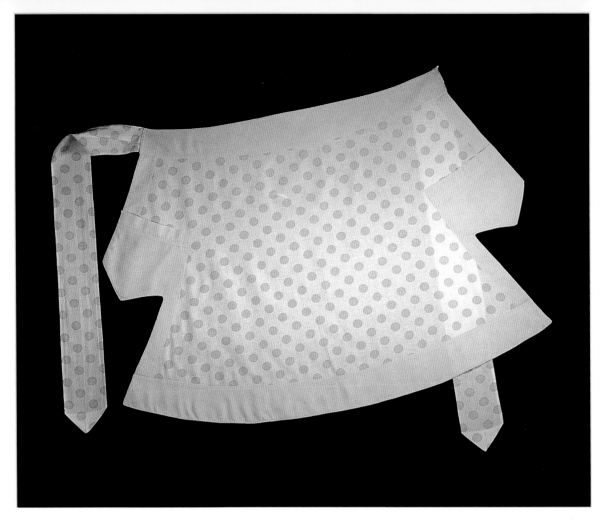

Two oddly-shaped **pentagonal side pockets** jut from the outer edges of this sunny yellow apron. Bold dime-size dots float on a flat field of white. The apron is framed by a wide band of solid yellow fabric, one inch along the sides and two and a half inches at the bottom. Can you locate the 'make-do' piecing?

Graceful curves and dainty dots are the main attraction here. An abundance of multicol-ored pea-size dots covers the apron. The drop-down waist, curved pocket, and lower edge are accented with decorative 'looped' red rickrack and bias binding.

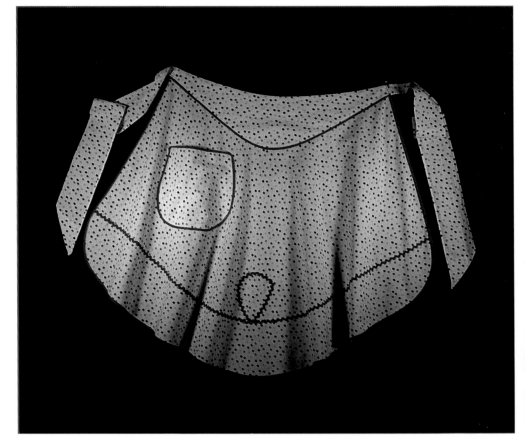

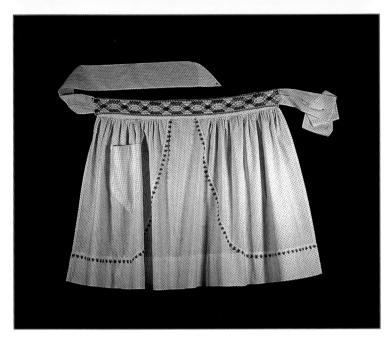

Miniature red dots lend a pinkish cast to this generously gathered apron. Call them micro or mini dots. Red and white trim in two sizes and styles is carefully applied to the waistband and skirt. The lower edge of the decorative trim is free (not stitched down). A V-shaped five-sided pocket has a fold-down upper edge.

What could be more attention-getting than this **vibrant and deeply pleated** red and white polka dot number? White lazy daisy flowers form a diamond pattern along the lower edge and highlight the patch pocket. Embroidery is by hand, with double-stranded white floss.

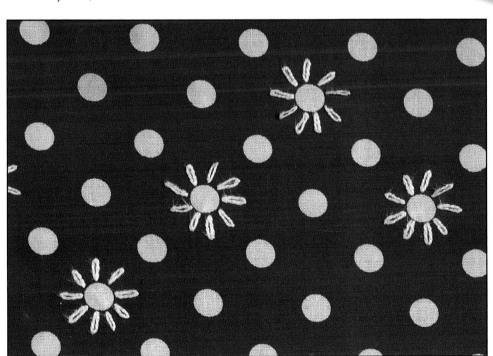

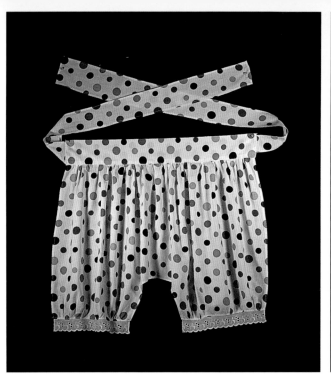
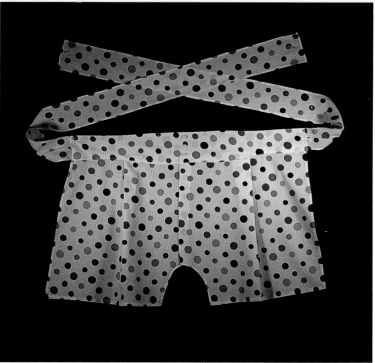

You might call it **the height (or depth) of apron kitsch**. The paired bloomers and boxers contrast gathers with pleats, and lace trim with a button fly. The fabric itself—multicolored multi-sized bubble gum-like balls—can hardly be taken seriously. A classic his and hers package, they are certain to elicit comments.

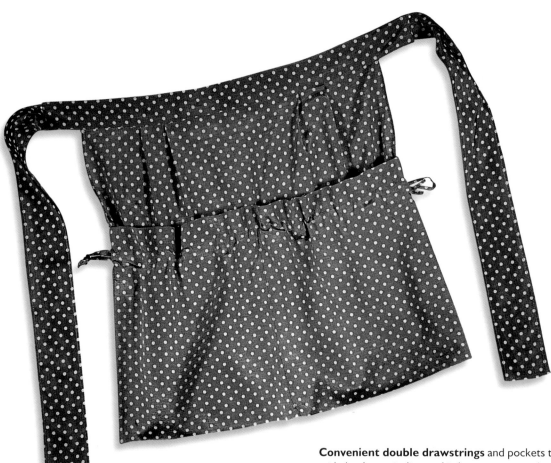

Convenient double drawstrings and pockets that are both deep and wide lend practicality to this lustrous gray and white polka dot design. The upper edge of this fabric blend apron has tiny pleats. Designed for temporary storage, it might have been used for clothespins, gathering garden produce, or toting needlework supplies.

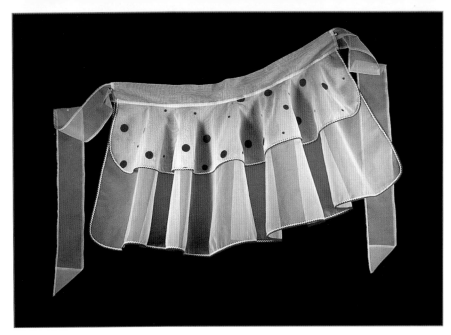

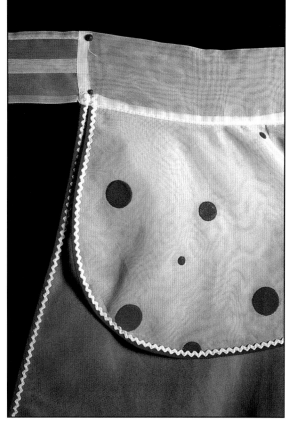

Sheer nylon organdy and **twelve feet of flounce** characterize this circular apron. Bright red mini and maxi dots float on the overskirt. All edges are rickracked and bound, and there is no pocket. Could this be the original *Dot Org* apron?

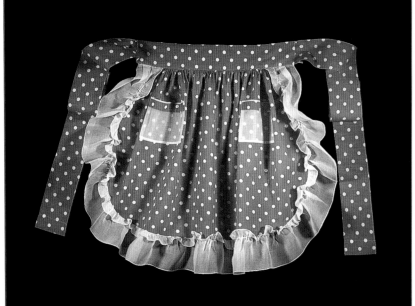

White organdy **double ruffles** add a stated feminine quality to this apron. One of the few that carries a commercial label ("Teatimer" by T-Time Apron Co., New York) it features a finely gathered waistline and extra long sashes. Decorative bands highlight the see-through pockets.

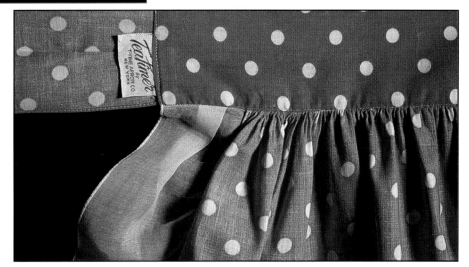

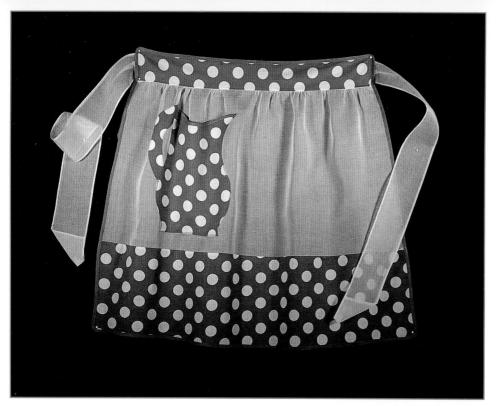

If you favor polka dots, you're sure to like this emerald green apron with the **nickel-sized white polka dots**. Adding to the drama is the nicely shaped water pitcher, which doubles as a generously deep pocket. The apron is outlined with green bias trim, and the sashes are 'P and P' style (pleated and pointed). The pocket is rather crudely appliquéd with machine zigzag stitches (some raw edges left revealed), and not likely to withstand rigorous laundering.

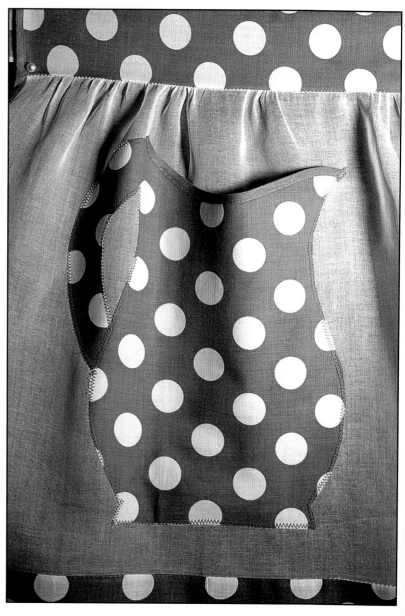

The Linear Look: Stripes and Plaids

A printed diagonal plaid with **aquamarine and acid green** will capture your attention on this one-piece cotton percale gathered apron. Its wide circular lower edge is contrasted with the rectangular pocket and stylized V-shaped waistband. Bright rickrack in two sizes edges the waistband, pocket, and lower edge.

Aprons in this section provide an antidote to the floral and polka dot patterns that prevail in the world of aprons. Look here for linear effects, whether vertical, horizontal, or diagonal. Allow the lines to carry your eyes through the parallels, perpendiculars, and zigzags that permeate the patterns.

Three categories of fabrics—stripes, plaids, and ginghams—make up the directional fabrics found on aprons. Stripes are easily defined as "textiles consisting of lines or bands against a plain background". The lines travel in one direction only. They may be printed or woven.

Plaids are "patterns of unevenly spaced repeated stripes crossing at right angles". The lines travel in both directions. These, too, may be printed or woven.

Ginghams are simply plaids with the same stripe running in both directions. By far, ginghams comprise the lion's share of directional fabrics appearing in aprons. However, only two unusual examples are included here. Numerous traditional gingham aprons are examined in greater detail in the previous section titled *Every Color Under the Sun*.

One ordinarily thinks of stripes and plaids as patterns that are *woven* into the fabric. It may come as a surprise that of the aprons included here, the majority are constructed from *printed* fabrics. Some of these are diagonally printed, e.g., the red and white checked apron and the turquoise and acid green plaid apron.

Both even and uneven plaids appear in these aprons. Some plaids are bold and wide repeat, others narrow and symmetrical. Some are matched with precision, others assembled with little or no thought to where and when the lines intersect each other. The gored apron with the zigzag effect is meticulously matched. In other aprons, some of the pockets have been precisely cut, e.g., the turquoise gingham/organdy. In contrast, some paired pockets don't even agree with each other, and most don't match the background to which they are applied.

As if to temper the straightforward and linear nature of the fabrics, several of these striped and plaid aprons have embellishments with softer lines and curves. Examples include gathered commercial lace, rickrack, scalloped edges, embroidery, and ruffles. Each lends a welcome and complementary relief to the rigidity of stripes and plaids.

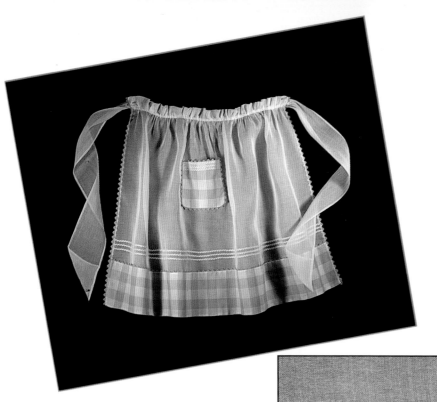

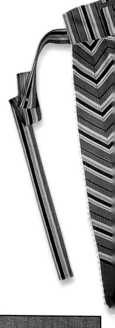

Inch wide turquoise gingham plaid is contrasted with sheer translucent organdy in this dressy serving apron. An unusual **ruffled waistline** is created by turning, gathering, and stitching the top of the apron. Rickrack in two colors and two sizes provides the accents. Delicate handmade feather stitches are used to apply the white rickrack on the pocket and border.

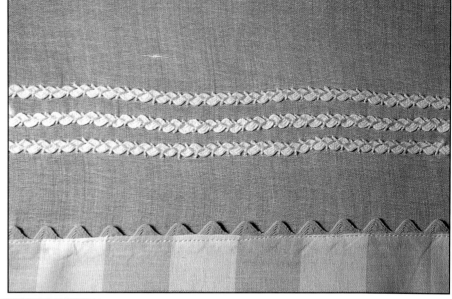

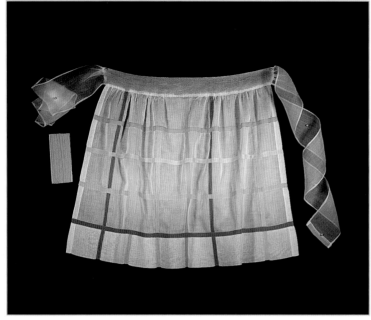

Half inch wide bias trim in pink, green, blue, and lavender creates **a plaid effect** on this gathered organdy apron. Horizontal and vertical lines are placed three inches apart and machine-stitched in place. No pocket on this purely decorative summery pastel design.

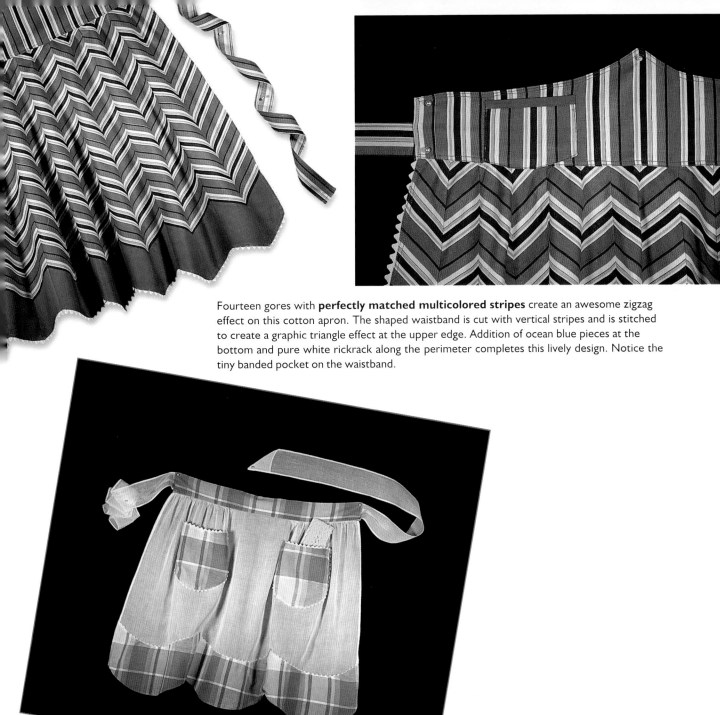

Fourteen gores with **perfectly matched multicolored stripes** create an awesome zigzag effect on this cotton apron. The shaped waistband is cut with vertical stripes and is stitched to create a graphic triangle effect at the upper edge. Addition of ocean blue pieces at the bottom and pure white rickrack along the perimeter completes this lively design. Notice the tiny banded pocket on the waistband.

A wide repeat woven plaid is paired with cotton organdy in this gathered apron. The well-rounded plaid pockets are trimmed with yellow rickrack. The gentle curves of **three large scallops** along the lower edge are also topped with rickrack. A person (or company) named Carmen Lee proudly included their label on the sash.

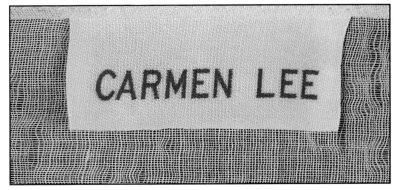

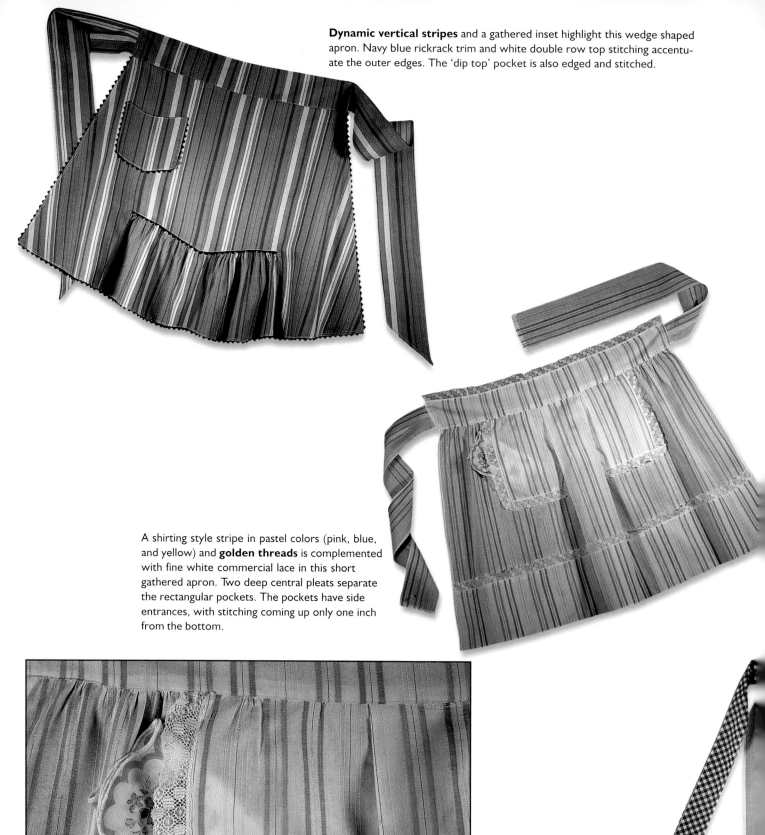

Dynamic vertical stripes and a gathered inset highlight this wedge shaped apron. Navy blue rickrack trim and white double row top stitching accentuate the outer edges. The 'dip top' pocket is also edged and stitched.

A shirting style stripe in pastel colors (pink, blue, and yellow) and **golden threads** is complemented with fine white commercial lace in this short gathered apron. Two deep central pleats separate the rectangular pockets. The pockets have side entrances, with stitching coming up only one inch from the bottom.

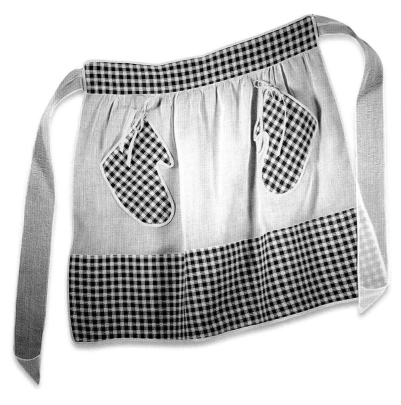

Cleverly shaped and placed **mitten pockets** with cheery yellow bows decorate this gathered organdy apron. All edges of this bright blue and yellow printed plaid are finished with narrow yellow bias trim. This design is certain to be noticed at any gathering. *An entire section of this book is devoted to pocket styles. Be sure to look there for additional imaginative designs.*

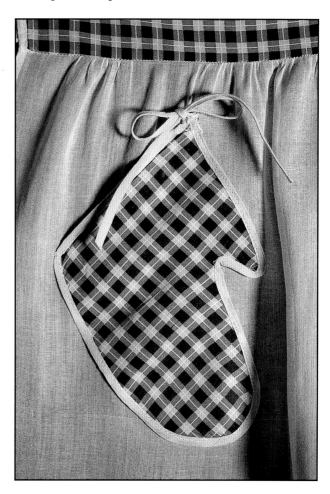

A hand embroidered **field of flowers** is the spotlight in this white organdy and red checkered apron. The 'mock' gingham is printed diagonally. The sashes are short, the pockets are square, and the flowers are delightful. "Lazy daisy" and "stem" are the embroidery stitches used.

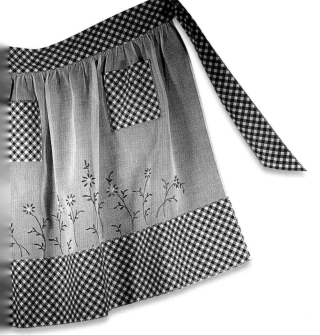

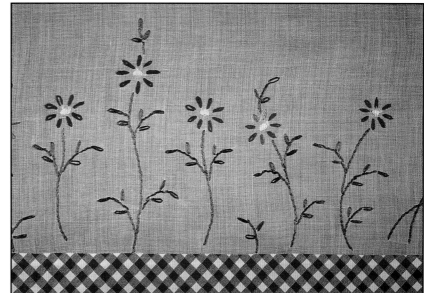

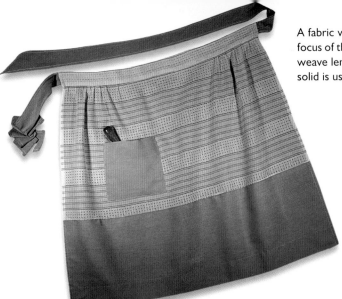

A fabric with blue pin stripes and delicate lacelike white are the focus of this gathered apron of **understated elegance**. The open weave lends an airy feeling to the upper portion. A periwinkle blue solid is used for the patch pocket, sashes, and lower portion.

Multi-colored vertical stripes draw the attention to this gathered short-sashed cotton apron. The stripes are complemented with rich blue solid fabric on the shaped waist, lower edge, and pentagonal pocket. Miniature white rickrack is used for trim. Not easily detected from the front is the built-in hot pad on the lower right corner. This five inch square is doubly padded and has an opening on its upper edge to insert the hand.

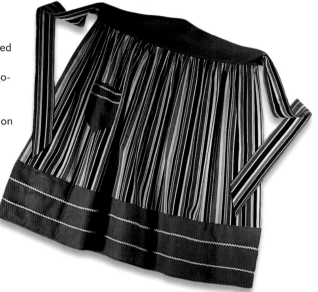

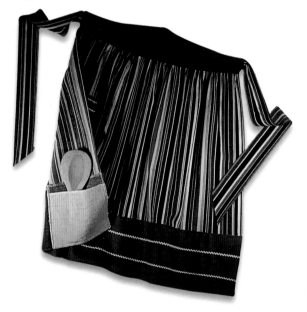

You'll need **twelve feet of pink and gold metallic rickrack** to complete this gathered circular wonder. White organdy and a pastel plaid of pink, gray, and turquoise team up in this unusual design. Notice how the sashes exit from the top of this apron, which has no waistband. No pocket either! Of what possible use could it be?

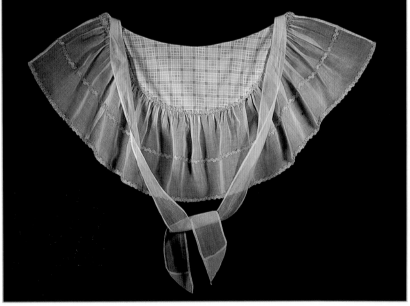

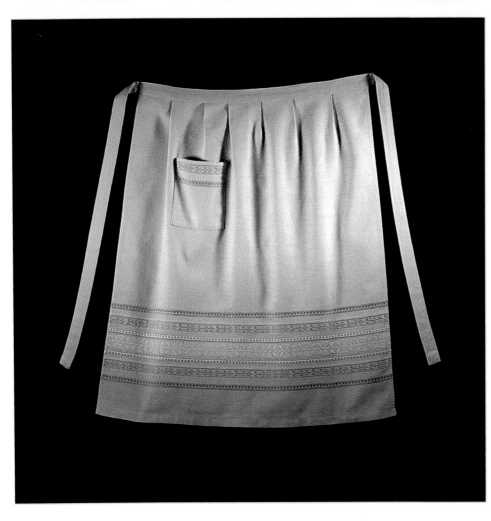

A five-inch-wide **machine woven border** in subtle pastels highlights the bottom of this sea foam green apron. Pink, yellow, blue, and white threads are woven into the symmetrical design, a portion of which also accents the rectangular pocket. Six tiny pleats and a combination waistband/sash top this apron of medium weight soft cotton fabric.

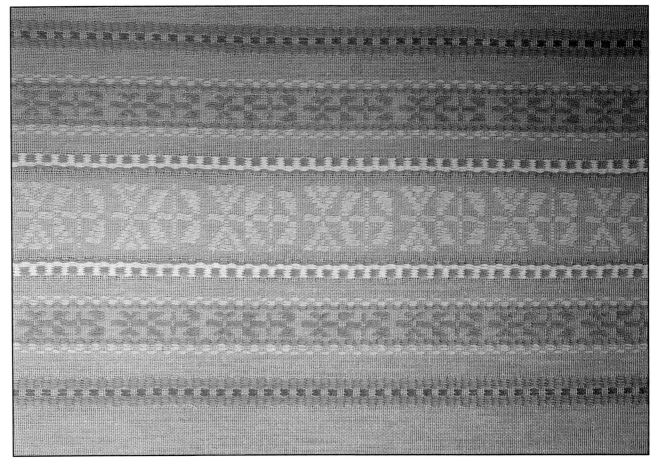

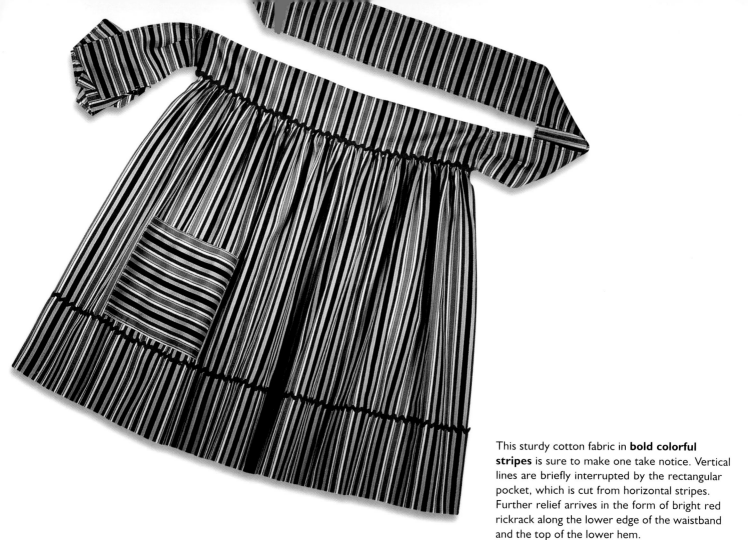

This sturdy cotton fabric in **bold colorful stripes** is sure to make one take notice. Vertical lines are briefly interrupted by the rectangular pocket, which is cut from horizontal stripes. Further relief arrives in the form of bright red rickrack along the lower edge of the waistband and the top of the lower hem.

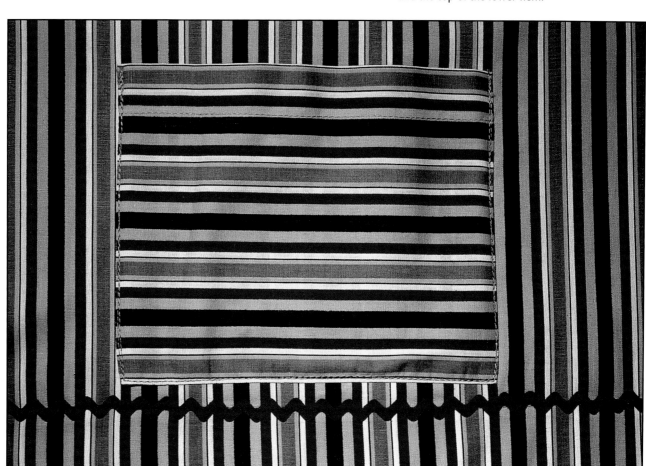

Section Two

ELEMENTS OF DESIGN

When Rickrack Was the Rage

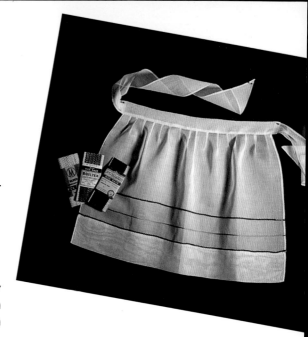

If the number of aprons edged and decorated with rickrack is any indication, the companies that produced and sold it during the mid-20th century must have done very well. Probably more aprons have it than don't. Yards and yards are required for some designs.

Rickrack was made of mercerized cotton fibers. It was machine washable, usually guaranteed color fast. One package proudly declared "Rick rack is one of the most suitable trimmings for all purposes—aprons, children's clothes, dresses, curtains." It further cautioned the user, "machine washable under commercial or home laundering conditions (do not boil or use bleaching agents). Dry away from direct sunlight." Additional claims such as "ironing never necessary," "no point curling," "wash 'n wear," "sta-flat," "unconditionally guaranteed for colorfastness and perfect workmanship" make it sound like an awesome product.

Several sizes were available, from the narrow miniature rickrack (about 1/8 inch wide) to the jumbo size (about 3/4 inch wide). Other sizes included 1/4 inch and 1/2 inch, which was the most frequently used. Narrow rickrack was commonly labeled Size 13, and was labeled "baby" rickrack by some companies. Half-inch wide rickrack had a 29 suffix—Size 29 or 429. Jumbo had a 45 suffix—Size 45, 445, 7145.

Some designers chose to use several sizes on one design. One of the white organdy aprons pictured in this section has a decorative border of three rows of red rickrack in three graduated sizes. Another fine example of graduated sizes is pictured in the *Pretty in Pink* section—a flared and frilly pink overskirted organdy apron with three rows of white rickrack in incremental sizes decorating both skirts.

The variety of colors available was like the rainbow, and more. Deep rich colors, bright primaries, pastels, tints, shades, and neutrals were among the choices. Packages were usually labeled by color name and/or number, e.g., canary 86, red 65, etc. Each package held from two to nine yards (higher amounts for the narrow styles).

The majority of designers chose to use only one style and color on their apron. One example in this section is the medium green gathered apron with the black rickrack zigzag border. This simple embellishment is very graphic. The rickrack is rather crudely applied, but oh-so-dramatic.

Employing the principle of repetition, the creator of the organdy and yellow floral apron has applied four identical horizontal rows of green rickrack. It makes a fine balance with the floral fabric, and, in fact, becomes the focal point of the design.

A **recycled cotton bag** was the starting point for this soft green loosely gathered apron. Black rickrack has been rather crudely hand stitched (in brown thread, no less) into an irregularly sharp zigzag design. The effect is very graphic and the apron is very practical.

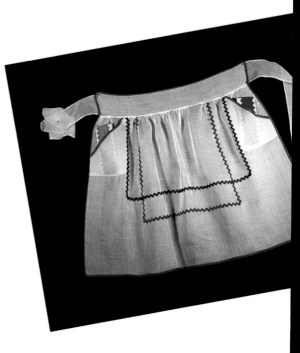

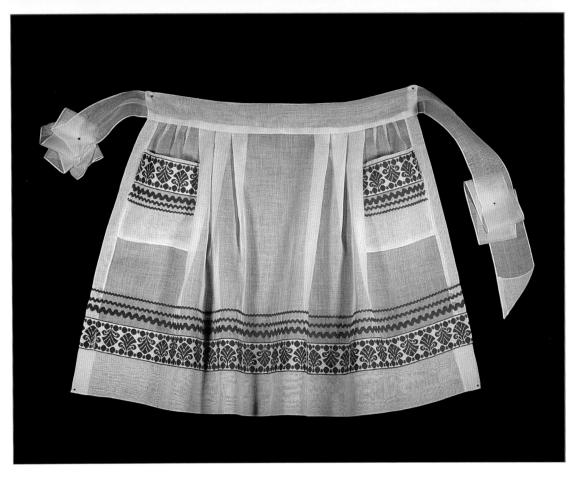

Rickrack in three companion sizes (1/8, 1/4, and 1/3 inch) and a two-inch band of scarlet trim embellish this pleated cotton apron. Paired pockets are similarly trimmed and inserted into the side hems.

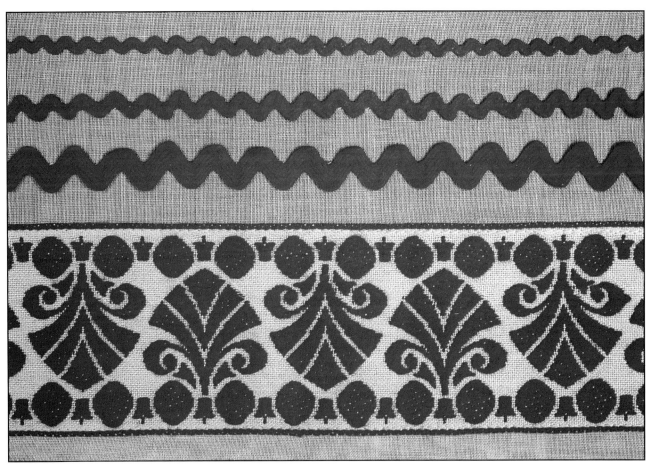

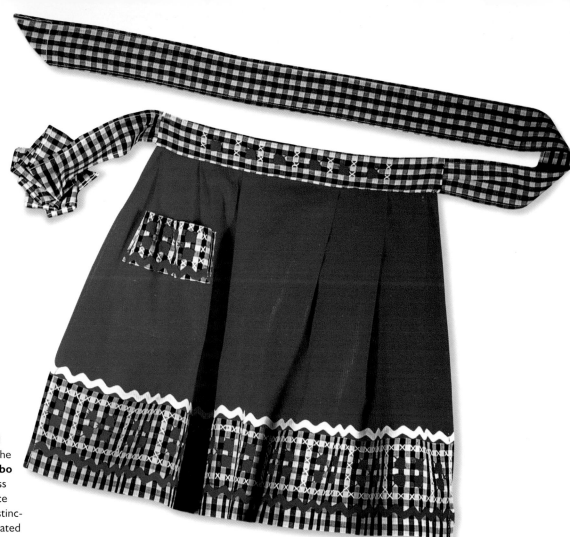

Black and white gingham and cherry red percale provide the background for 3/4 inch **jumbo rickrack**. Sizable white cross stitches and red Teneriffe lace designs make a border of distinction, parts of which are repeated on the pocket and waistband.

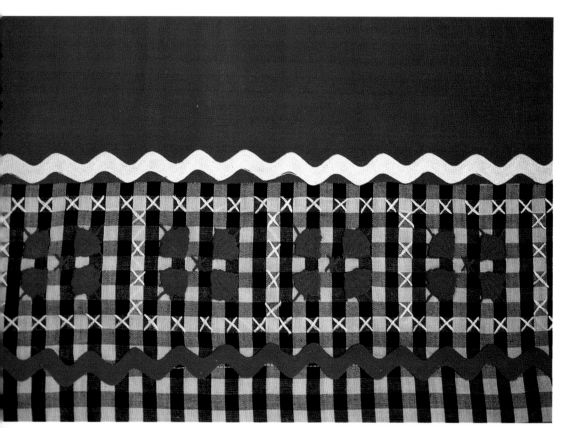

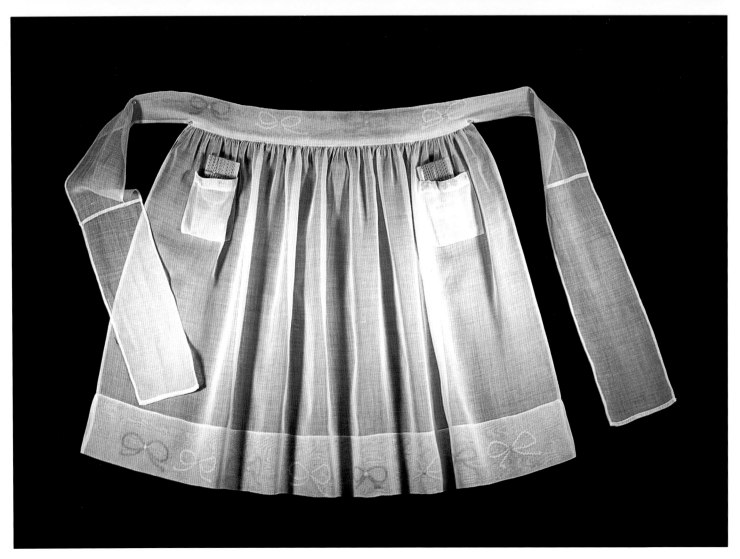

A very attractive and unique shadow effect is created on this gathered white apron. **Miniature rickrack bows** have been shaped and inserted between layers of organdy. Four three-inch bows in pink, yellow, green, and blue have been hand tacked in the waistband, eight bows in the lower hem. The centers of the bows are accented with contrasting embroidery thread. The waistband and sash are constructed in combination, with extensions. Tiny bows (each about one inch wide) appear in the upper band of each pocket.

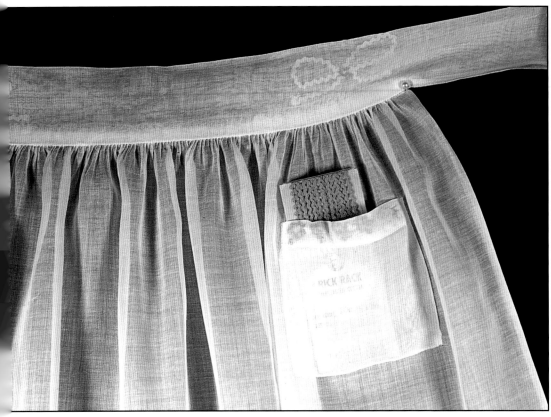

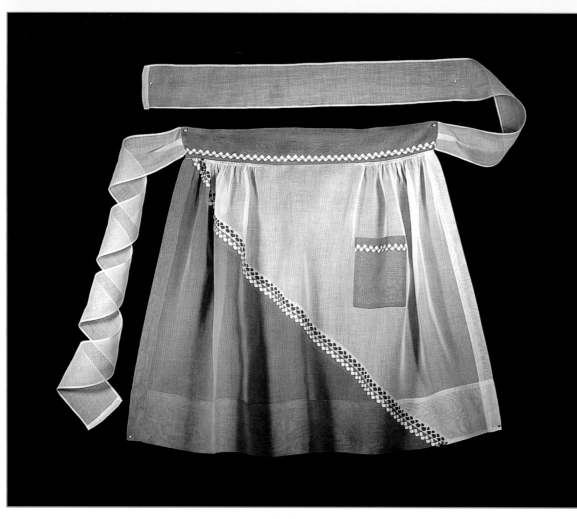

Snowy white and emerald green prevail on this gathered organdy apron. Parallel rows of green and white rickrack straddle the diagonal seam and are anchored with hand stitched contrasting embroidery thread. Rickrack also accents the waistband and pocket of this dramatic design.

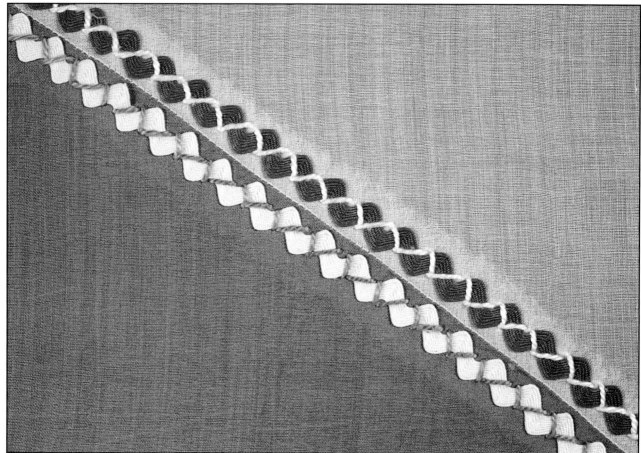

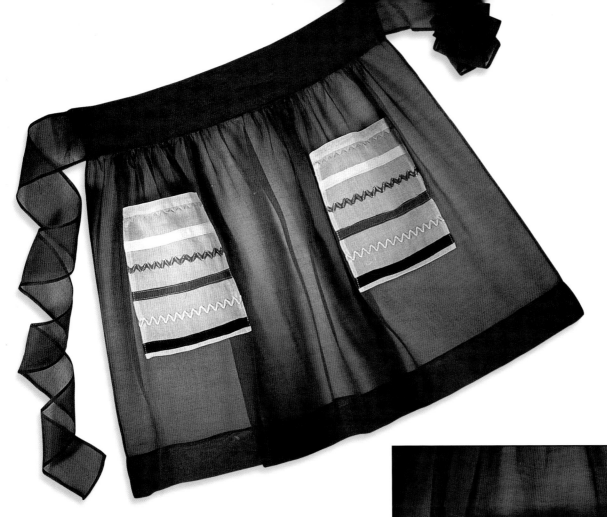

Three styles of rickrack decorate the yellow rectangular pockets of this chocolate brown gathered design. The upper pocket edge is trimmed with light turquoise rickrack, the center has gold metallic threads woven into dark green, and the bottom has a dual color turquoise and white design. The machine-stitched bands of white, brown, and navy blue are half inch strips of organdy.

Needle Arts:
Embroidery, Crochet, Tatting, Lace

The aprons in this chapter represent a real mixed bag of decorative needle arts. Most prominent are the examples of six genre: cross stitch, embroidery, Swedish 'huck' weaving, crochet, tatting, and lace. The techniques of appliqué and piecing are also considered needle arts. However, they are more significantly structural than decorative techniques and are explored in the chapter titled *Pieced and Appliquéd*.

Cross stitch appears to be the most common form of hand needlework on aprons. However, you won't find many examples in this chapter. Cross stitched designs are mainly associated with gingham checked aprons. These are also treated separately and at length in a chapter called *Every Color Under The Sun*.

The sole example of a cross stitch design in this section is on a nongingham loosely woven yellow cotton apron. The stitches are very small (about eleven X's per inch), far smaller than the cross stitches customarily found on gingham aprons. Standard woven ginghams are eight checks per inch, others wider at four checks per inch. In these instances, the X's occur at eight per inch (standard cross stitching) and four per inch (sometimes referred to as 'chicken scratching'), respectively. So the example included here is much more intricate in design and detail.

Hand embroidery is another widespread needle art technique applied to aprons. From pastoral scenes to holiday themes, embroidery is the ubiquitous medium for depiction of ideas and details. Floral patterns are especially popular, and several well-executed designs are pictured here.

If you are an embroidery aficionado, be on the alert for other designs scattered throughout the book, including several good examples in the *Children's Aprons* section.

A graphic example of Swedish 'huck' weaving is also included. This modified method of embroidery is usually done on huck toweling (hence the name), or in some cases, on dotted organdy or dotted Swiss. Both of these fabrics have a raised surface (of threads or dots) onto which the stitches are attached. Swedish weaving is really a darning technique, straight running stitches between two points. Nothing fancy or difficult to execute. Even more basic than cross stitching. Beautiful patterns are created by stitching from point to point with embroidery floss in a color contrasting to the background.

A lovely turquoise on white dotted organdy apron is pictured. Three additional aprons with Swedish weaving are included elsewhere in the book. Other dotted organdy designs can be found in the *Polka Dot* and *Seeing Red* sections. Also, peek in the *Pretty in Pink* section for an apron made with *real* huck toweling.

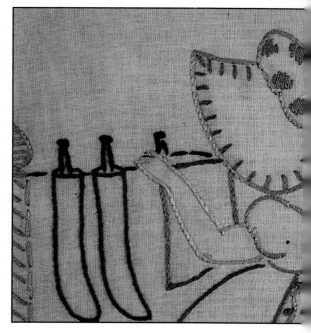

An **aproned and bonneted** lass clearly portrays the purpose for this utilitarian clothespin apron. Durable unbleached muslin is cutaway into deep dual entry pockets and bound with red bias tape. This apron was made from a prestamped kit or transferred design. Embroidery stitches include stem, running, satin, and French knot.

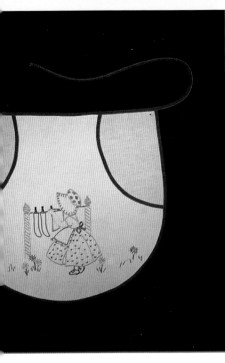

Three examples of aprons with crocheted designs or edging are pictured. One design method involves application of crocheted designs to the skirt of the apron and cutting away the background fabric. Another method uses a substantial crocheted design along the upper edge of the apron and on the pocket. A third more common method is to decorate the perimeter with hand-crocheted edging.

Two of the crocheted examples are particularly impressive because they are white-on-white. One is sheer cotton organdy, the other lightweight cotton batiste. Without the distraction of color, the eye is free to examine and admire the design and stitching details of the crocheted pattern.

Two aprons with tatted edging are pictured. Tatting is one of the oft-neglected and under-appreciated needle arts. Most people are unable to identify it. Others have only heard of it. Still others have a bit of awareness because they had a mother or grandmother who did it. Very few people know how to do it. Very few *living* people, anyway.

Both aprons have tatted edging around the perimeter and on the pocket. The similarities end there. One is lightweight white fabric with an intricate 3/4 inch wide tatted edge. In contrast, the other apron is dark navy with a narrow 1/8 inch bright red tatted edge.

A lone example of an apron embellished with lace is also included. It was pur-

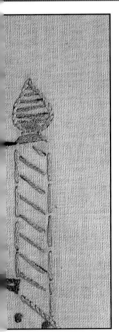

chased in a vintage linens shop in Munich, Germany. That alone makes it special. The intricate red and white hand worked lace that accents the waistband and lower edge makes it extra special.

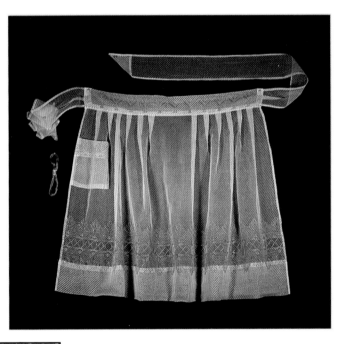

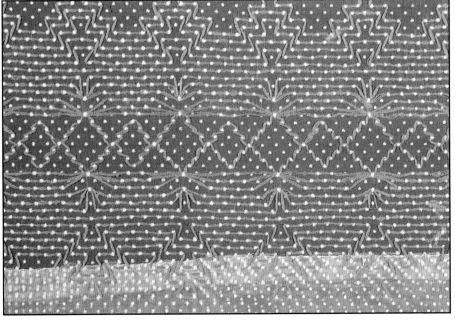

Elaborate **Swedish 'huck' weaving** has converted plain white dotted organdy into an apron of elegant design. Turquoise embroidery thread is stitched in dot-to-dot fashion for a six-inch mirror-image border. Carefully placed accents are stitched on the pocket and waistband. Note how the pocket hugs the outer edge.

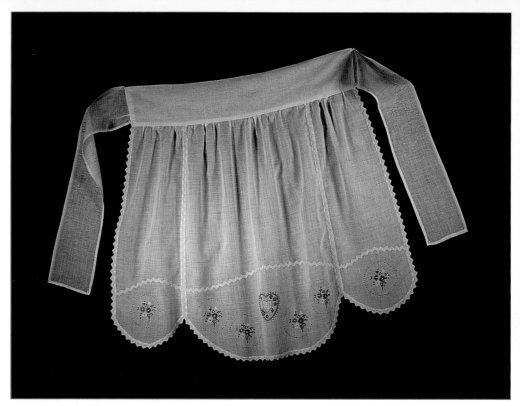

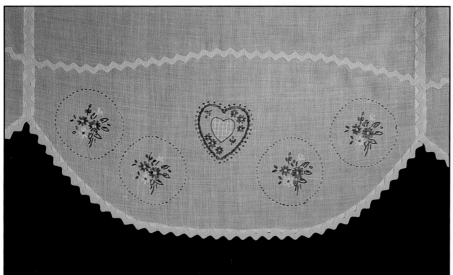

Soft, sheer, and delicate are words to describe this embroidered cotton lawn apron. Six floral bouquets encircled in green running stitches and one heart motif adorn the lower edge. Gently angled lines of hand appliquéd yellow rickrack frame the needlework and outer edges. Note the unusually wide (3 1/4 inches) waistband. All seams and edges on the reverse side are painstakingly double turned and hand stitched.

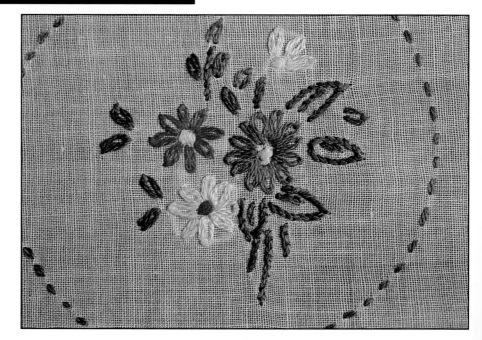

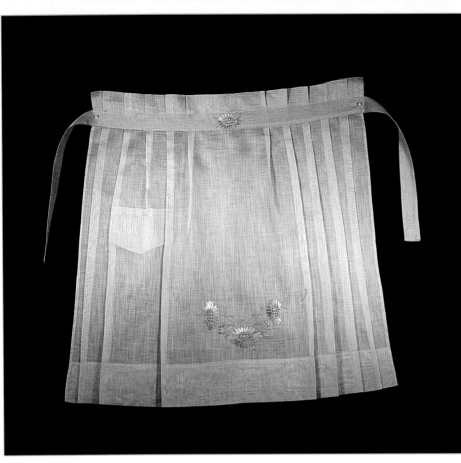

Precise pleats and elegant embroidery are the focus of this twilight blue organdy apron. Six-stranded variegated pink and three-stranded green floss make up the rich floral arrangement. Golden French knots form the center clusters. The ten half-inch pleats are covered and top stitched with a one-piece waistband and sashing.

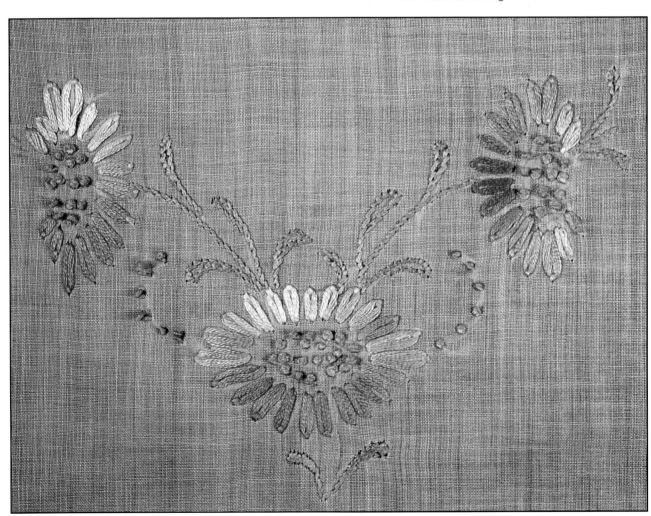

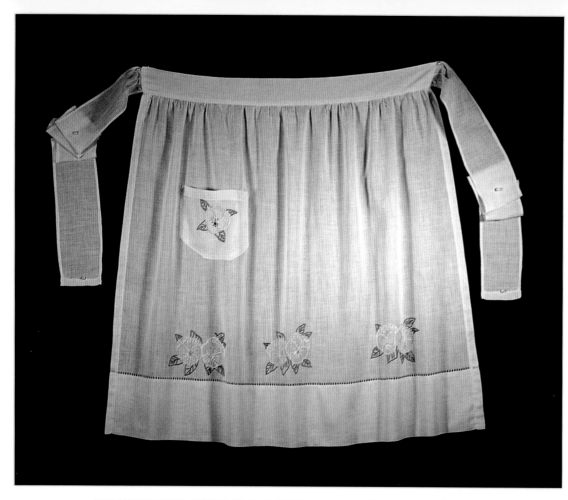

Baby blue batiste fabric is the background for pastel pansies embroidered in pink, white, and yellow. Leaves and details are stitched in green. The wide hexagonal pocket boasts a variegated pansy. A narrow (1/8 inch) pulled thread border tops the four-inch hem. Several horizontal threads have been removed, and the remaining vertical threads have been grouped with fine hem stitching.

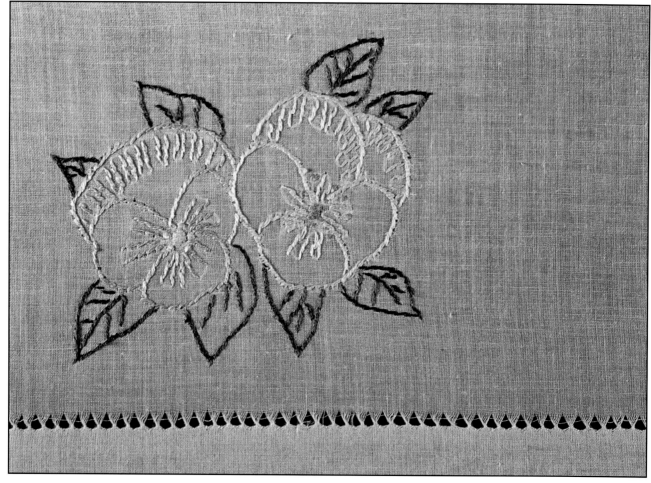

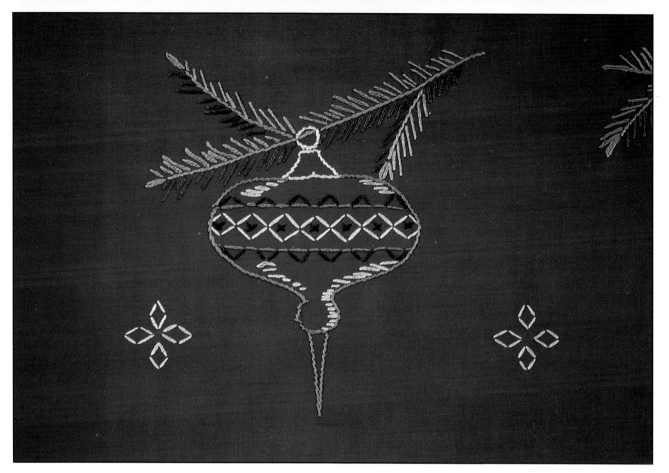

This cherry red gathered apron might put you **in the holiday spirit**. Hand-embroidered ornaments hang from pine boughs wrought in two shades of green. Detailed designs in two shades of blue and white decorate each ornament, and snowflakes float in the background.

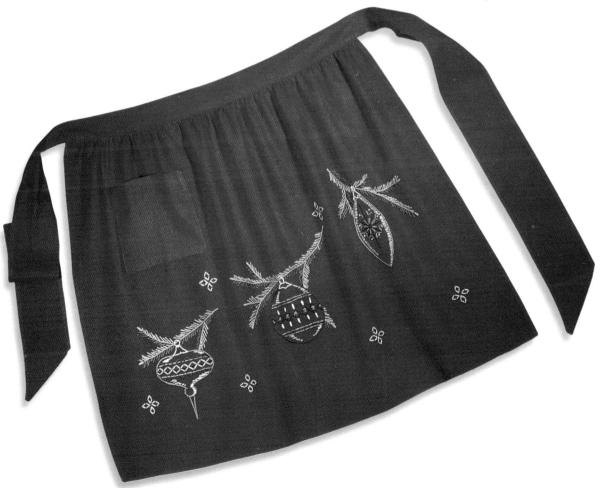

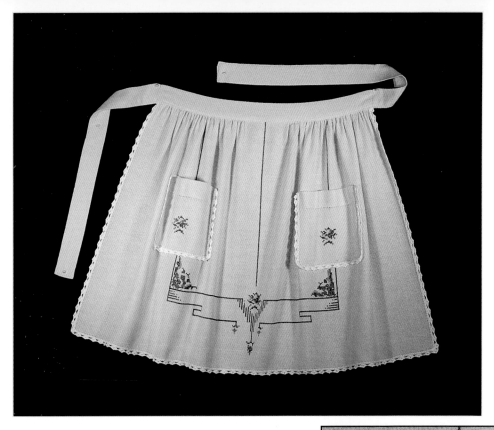

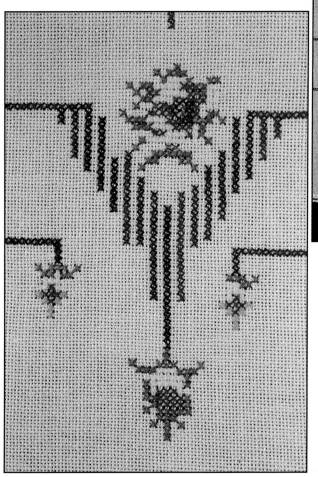

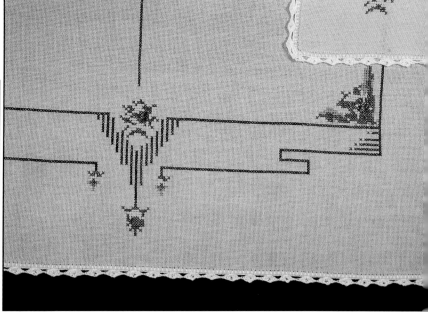

A **sunshine yellow cotton** is the perfect backdrop for these miniature cross stitch designs. Coarsely woven threads form a grid work for the classic lines in variegated brown and bronze. Floral clusters contribute to the art deco look. The pockets and apron perimeter are finished with white hand-crocheted edging.

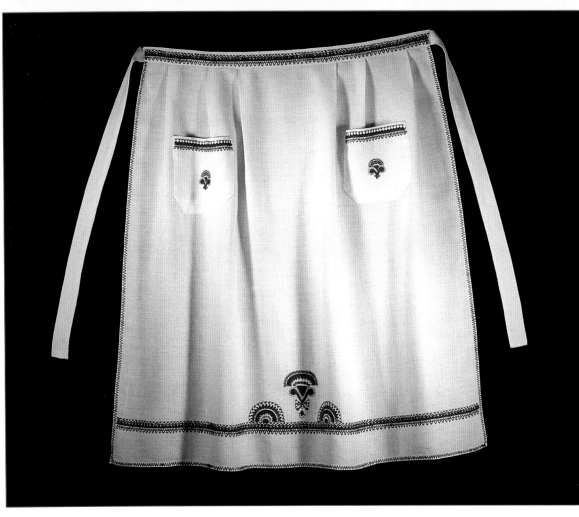

Flawless embroidery in deep scarlet and black on softly pleated creamy white linen marks this as among the most exquisite of aprons. The upper and lower bands (each 3/4 inch wide) are composed of five separately stitched narrow designs. Perfectly executed radiating designs lend an ethnic flavor. Miniature designs and bands grace the hexagonal pockets.

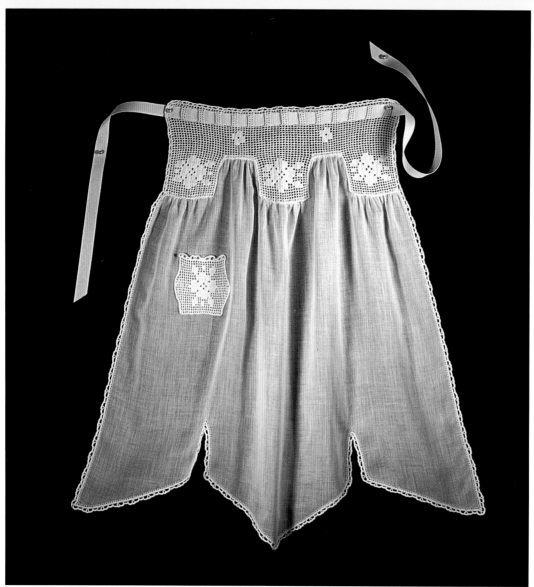

Sheer cotton batiste is combined with **delicate crocheted lace** for this dainty all-white apron. The crocheted upper edge has provision for an interwoven grosgrain ribbon sash (freshly replaced). The upper edge is lightly gathered and the lower edge is deeply notched and finished with crochet trim. The slightly rounded wee pocket (about three inches in each direction) claims its own crocheted edging.

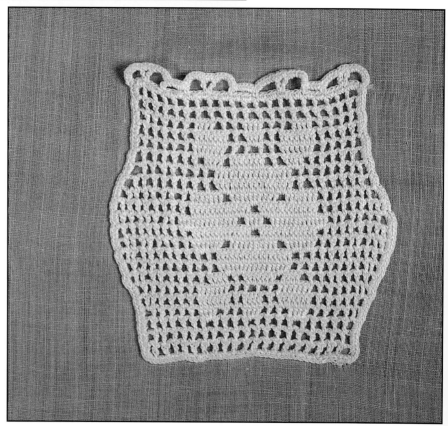

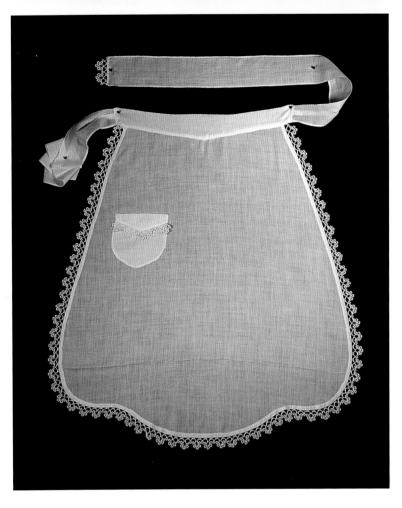

Intricate tatting is the eye catcher in this pear-shaped apron. Fine windowpane cotton has become even finer with use and laundering. Wear is especially evident on the ends of the sashes. The U-shaped mock flap pocket is also edged with the showy 3/4-inch tatting.

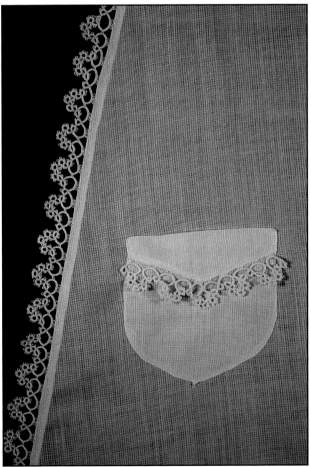

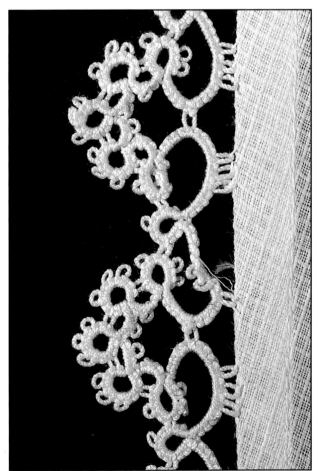

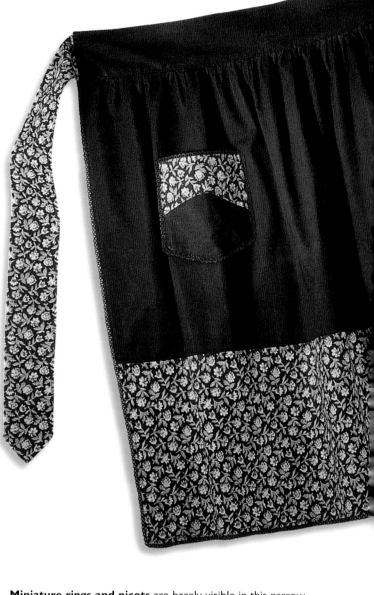

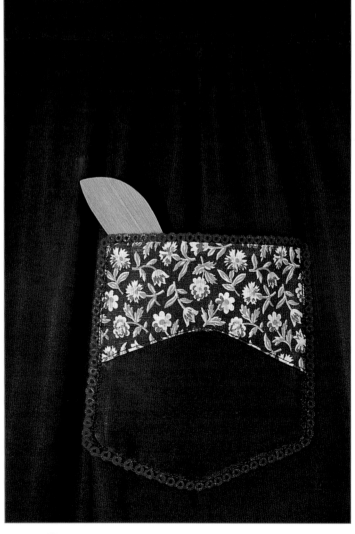

Miniature rings and picots are barely visible in this narrow (3/16 inch) red edging. Tatting could hardly be finer. The deep indigo gathered apron is further enhanced with a fine floral calico on the lower edge, sashes, and pocket.

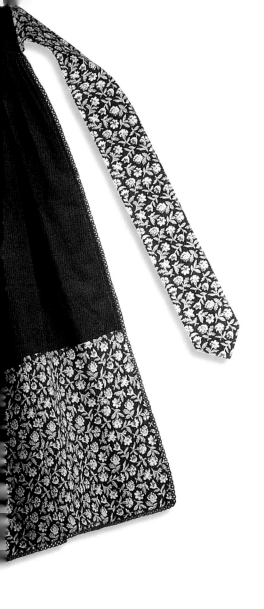

Hand-crocheted butterflies in two patterns drift across this lovely white-on-white translucent cotton organdy apron. The delicate broad-winged insects have been hand appliquéd and the background fabric has been cut away. A narrow waistband, a deep hem, and a rounded pocket complete the design.

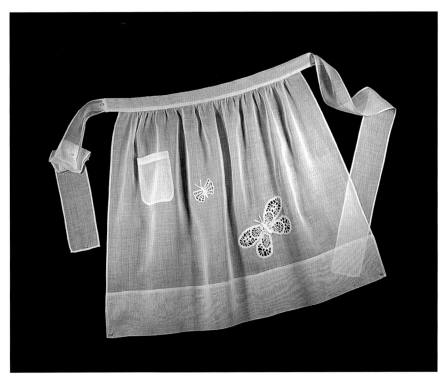

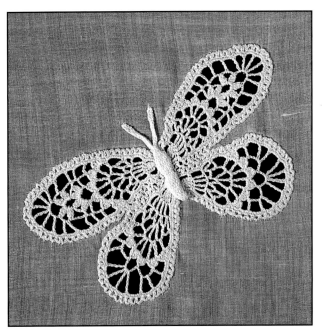

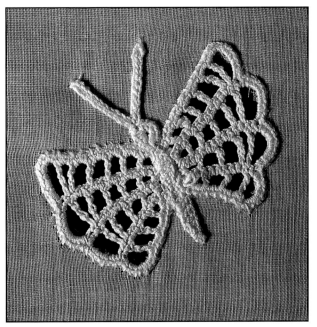

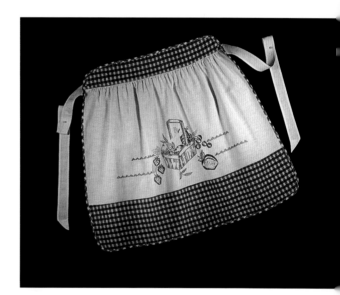

This elongated **linen and lace** apron has its own international flavor. A five-inch wide red and white band of lace with elegant birds and flowers graces the lower edge. The bird pattern is also stitched to the waistband, which is secured with two large hooks and eyes. This apron was purchased in a resale shop in Munich, Germany.

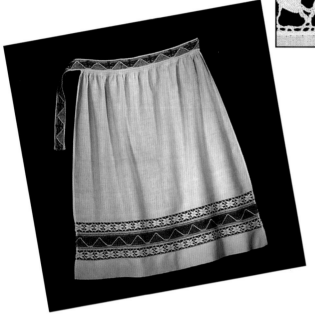

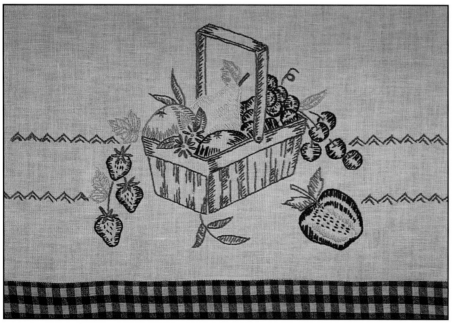

A basket overflowing with fruit makes **a delicious arrangement** on this sturdy unbleached muslin and red checked apron. All the apples, pears, oranges, cherries, grapes, and strawberries are hand-embroidered. The designs were transferred from a pattern, and the lightly gathered and bias bound apron was preassembled. From the collection of Lucy Bauer; hand embroidery by her mother, Della Macomber.

Pieced and Appliquéd

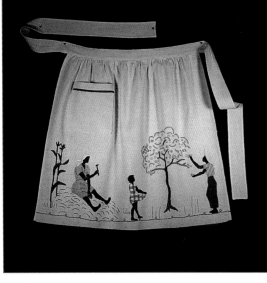

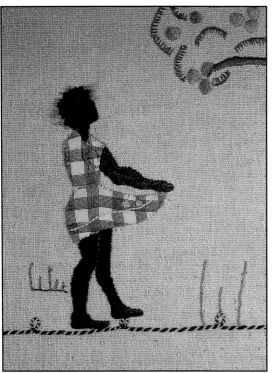

The gathering of the harvest dominates this **appliquéd and embroidered** tropical scene. The fruit-laden tree is stitched with satin and blanket stitches, and articles of clothing are hand-appliquéd to the beige flecked coarse cotton fabric. Dark green accents the pocket and lower edge. The looped horizontal lower dark red line is attached with yellow couching stitches.

Aprons in this section incorporate the two main staples of the quilting world—piecing and appliqué. In *pieced* designs, many small pieces are cut from fabrics and stitched in seams with right sides together. In *appliquéd* designs, shapes are cut from another cloth and laid on or applied to the top of the fabric. In either case, stitching may be done by hand or machine.

Piecing is a technique that creates the substance of the item. Although its primary role is a structural one, it will also become part of the design and decoration. Familiar geometric shapes are commonly used. The pieced aprons shown here are comprised mainly of squares, rectangles, and triangles in a range of sizes.

The most unusual pieced patterns are found on the Seminole aprons. The size and number of pieces, the vast range of colors, and the extravagant rickrack embellishments surpass any other apron in the book. The makers clearly pulled out all the stops on these aprons, and the piecing *has* become the design.

In contrast, appliqué is usually a decorative technique. It requires a background fabric (structure) on which shapes are applied. Appliquéd pieces are turned under at the edges, laid onto the background fabric, and stitched into place. It is usually more time consuming than piecing and requires more skill.

The appliquéd aprons pictured here range from those with numerous extremely tiny pieces to those with very large, even huge cutout shapes. You will discover wee flower petals and leaves skillfully arranged in floral bouquets and secured with microscopic hand stitches. You will also find larger-than-life tulips anchored with machine stitches and immense violets affixed with blanket stitches. And you will find one 'shadow appliqué' floral cutout behind a veil of dark navy blue.

Many appliquéd aprons suggest a subject or theme, e.g., a specific holiday, a season (springtime, harvest, or winter), a card party. Prominently appliquéd designs may become the center of attention on the apron and can dictate, even limit, its use.

There is as much variety among the examples of appliquéd aprons as any others in the entire book. Some of the prettiest and most picturesque designs can be found here.

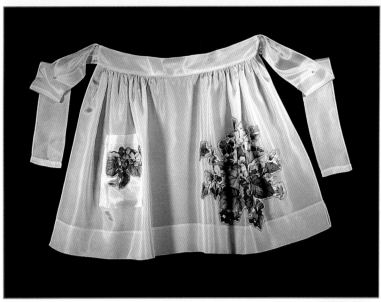

Festive clusters of violets become the centerpiece of this rayon taffeta gathered apron. A blanket stitch in purple thread outlines the floral arrangements. A smaller decal floats on the patch pocket. The edges of the floral fabric have not been turned under.

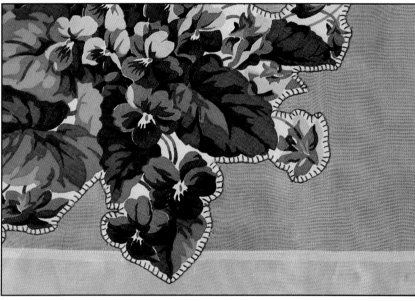

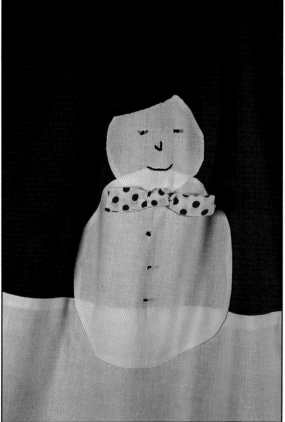

A **top-hatted and bow-tied** snow person appears to be looking for companions on this crimson and white gathered apron. French-knotted black buttons and eyes are among the minimal details on this well-rounded figure.

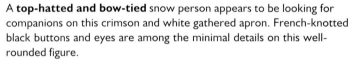

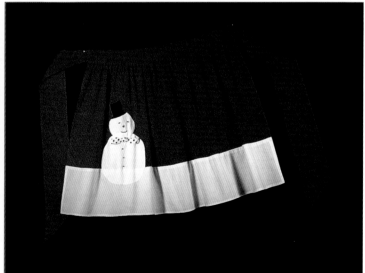

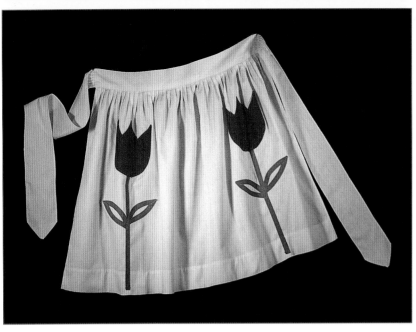

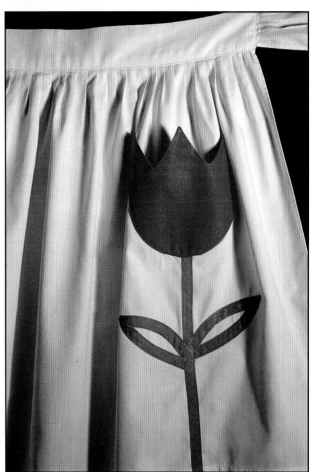

Showy red tulips with bright green stems and leaves have been machine appliquéd and **transformed into pockets** on this cheery yellow apron. Each pocket is fully lined, and the waistband is stitched into a rhythmic row of petite pleats.

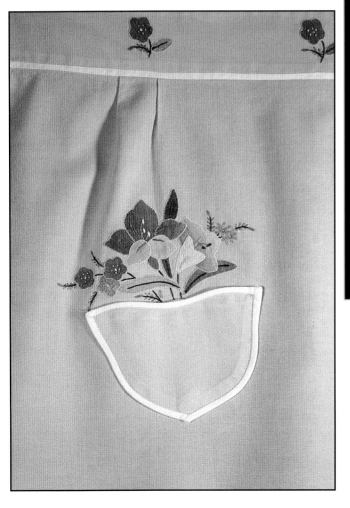

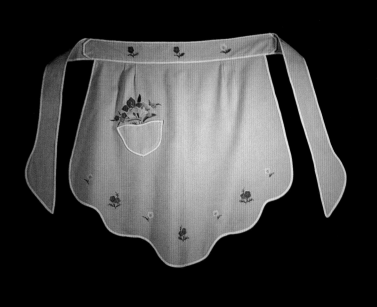

The fine art of appliqué is clearly evident in this mint-green apron of floral arrangements. A tinted and shaded bouquet emerges from the pocket, and single and paired blooms embellish the lower edge and waistband. Details are hand-embroidered and all edges are neatly bound in white. The waistband ends are carefully cornered and the sash ends are gently rounded.

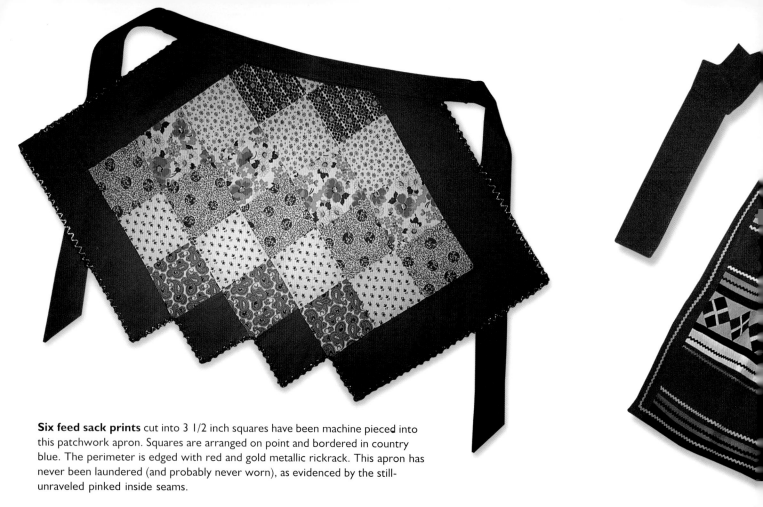

Six feed sack prints cut into 3 1/2 inch squares have been machine pieced into this patchwork apron. Squares are arranged on point and bordered in country blue. The perimeter is edged with red and gold metallic rickrack. This apron has never been laundered (and probably never worn), as evidenced by the still-unraveled pinked inside seams.

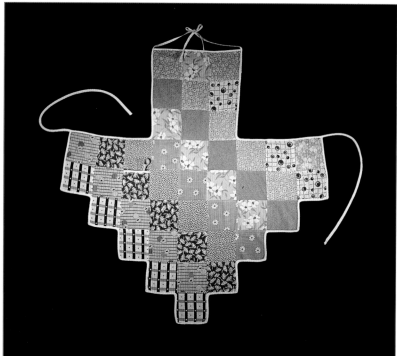

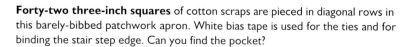

Forty-two three-inch squares of cotton scraps are pieced in diagonal rows in this barely-bibbed patchwork apron. White bias tape is used for the ties and for binding the stair step edge. Can you find the pocket?

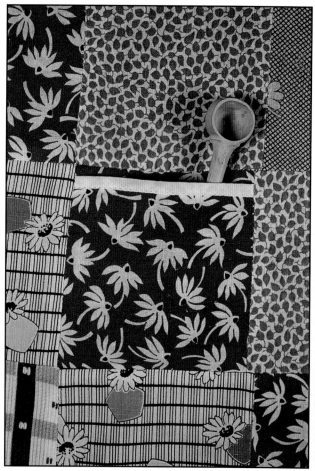

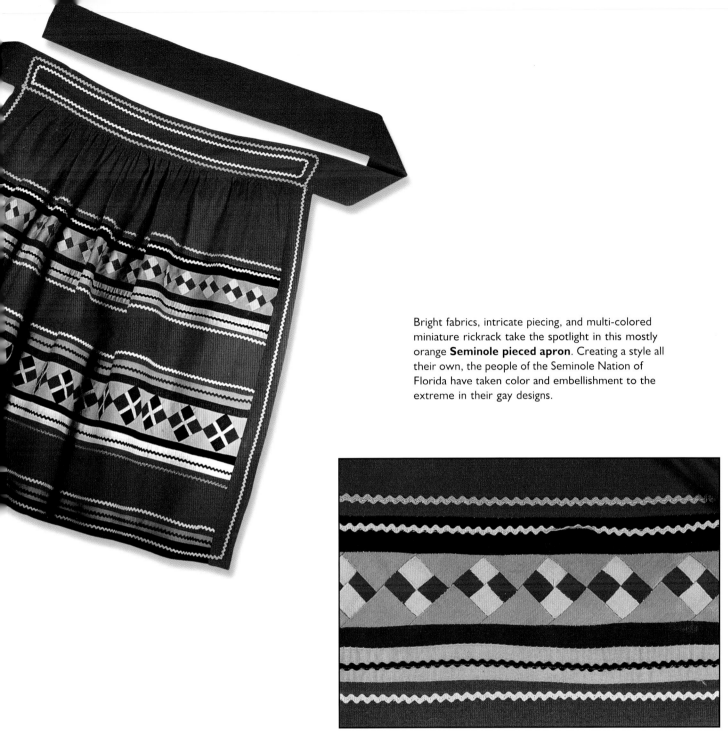

Bright fabrics, intricate piecing, and multi-colored miniature rickrack take the spotlight in this mostly orange **Seminole pieced apron**. Creating a style all their own, the people of the Seminole Nation of Florida have taken color and embellishment to the extreme in their gay designs.

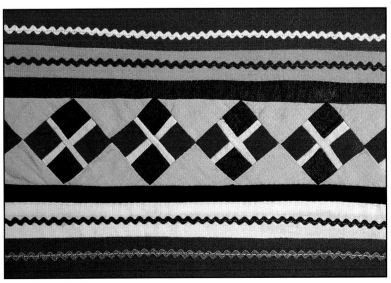

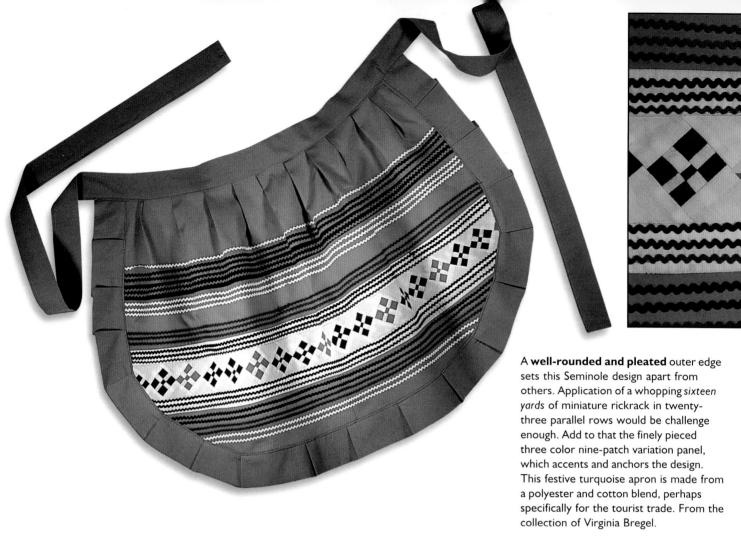

A **well-rounded and pleated** outer edge sets this Seminole design apart from others. Application of a whopping *sixteen yards* of miniature rickrack in twenty-three parallel rows would be challenge enough. Add to that the finely pieced three color nine-patch variation panel, which accents and anchors the design. This festive turquoise apron is made from a polyester and cotton blend, perhaps specifically for the tourist trade. From the collection of Virginia Bregel.

Lavender and purple flowered fabric with a touch of greenery and soft yellow cotton have been cut into three inch squares for this patch-work apron. Forty-one squares have been **set on point** and machine pieced checkerboard style. The upper edge has been stitched to a combination waistband/sash. The lower stair step border and angled sides are trimmed with white rickrack. The miniature pocket (same size as the pieces in the apron) is placed on edge and rickracked on all sides.

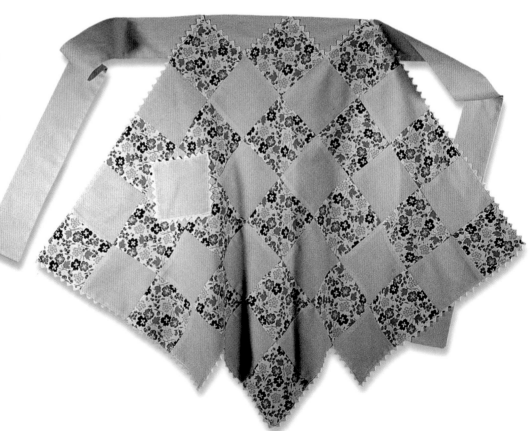

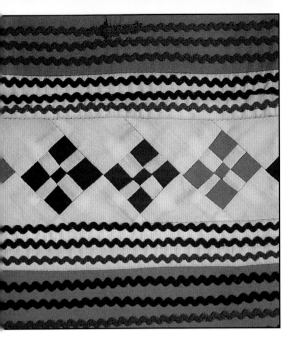

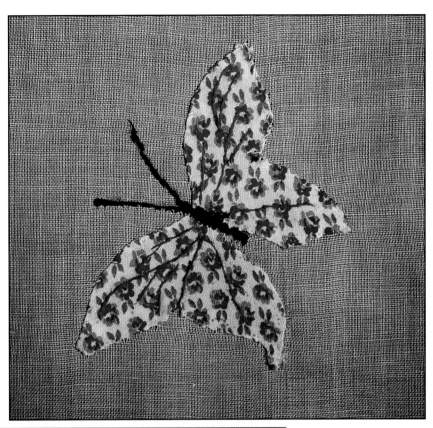

A solitary butterfly makes its way to a bouquet of showy raspberry red roses on this gathered white organdy apron. All details are hand appliquéd. The large rose has been modified into a pocket, complete with a lining and upper edge opening. Anatomical details on the butterfly are stem stitched with black embroidery floss. Did you notice the pieced extensions on the sashes?

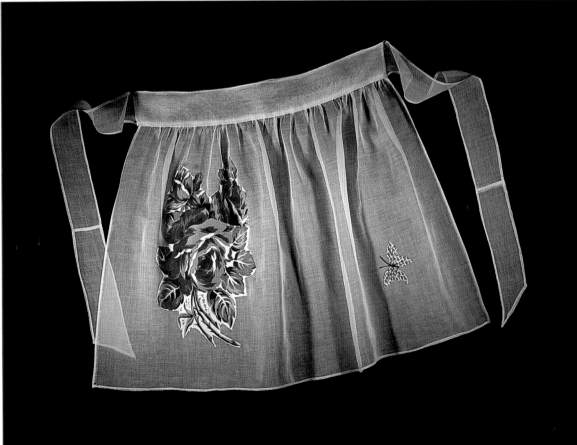

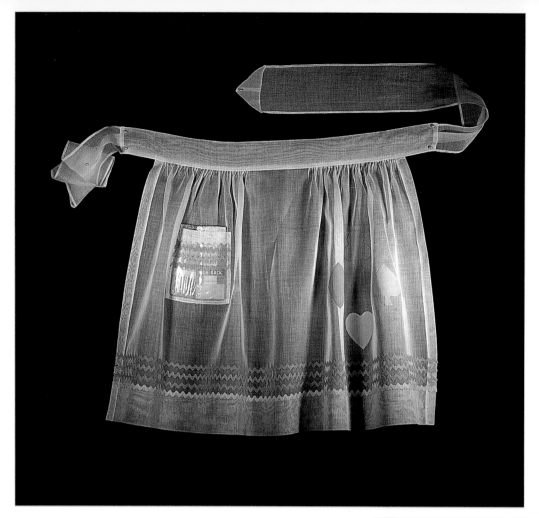

The hostess will be **properly attired** and prepared for an afternoon of playing cards in this sheer organdy apron. Four parallel rows of rickrack in pastel pink, yellow, green, and blue form a parade across the lower edge and pocket. A club, a spade, a heart, and a diamond in coordinated colors are hand-appliquéd on the skirt.

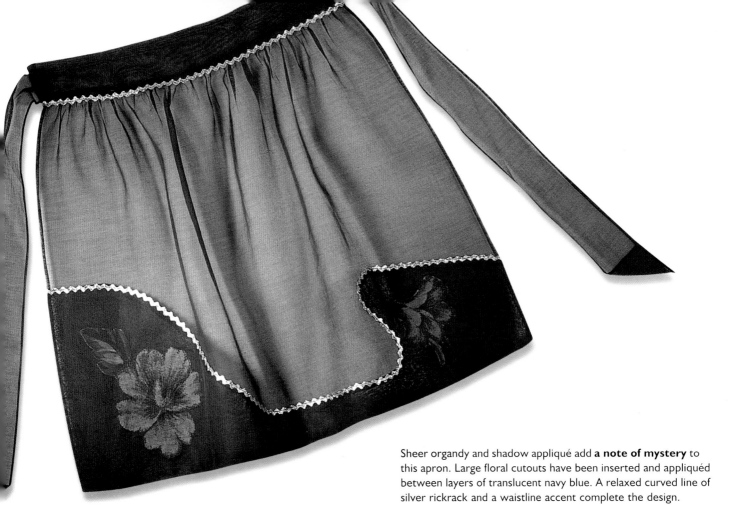

Sheer organdy and shadow appliqué add **a note of mystery** to this apron. Large floral cutouts have been inserted and appliquéd between layers of translucent navy blue. A relaxed curved line of silver rickrack and a waistline accent complete the design.

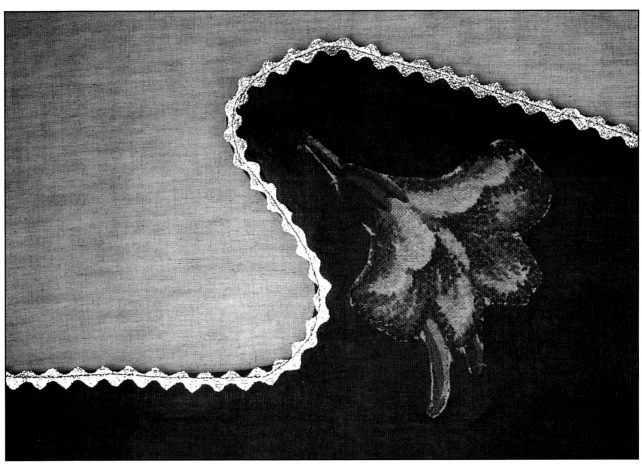

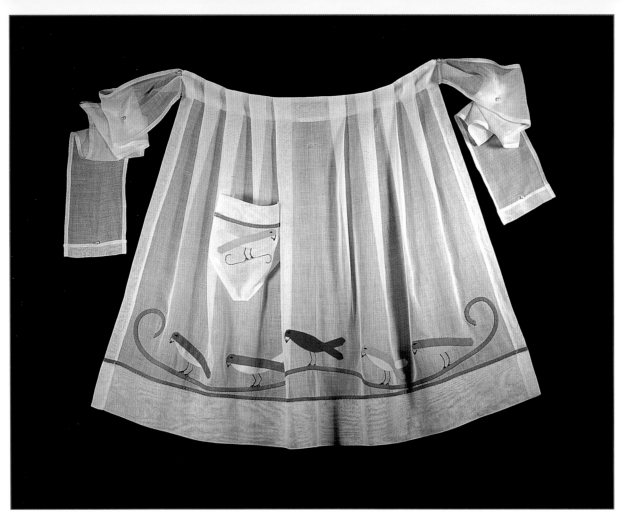

Assorted colorful **feathered friends** sit perched on a vine of greenery on this organdy apron. Each bird is a finely hand-appliquéd two-tone composition with a broad beak, skinny legs, and an eye (and eyebrow) embroidered in black. Eight one-inch pleats radiate from the center top, which is faced with organdy (no separate waistband). The six-sided pocket has an oddly narrow base and wide upper hem. The horizontal green trim at the top of the hem and pocket is *machine* zigzagged, in seeming contradiction to the *hand* appliquéd greenery on which the birds are perched.

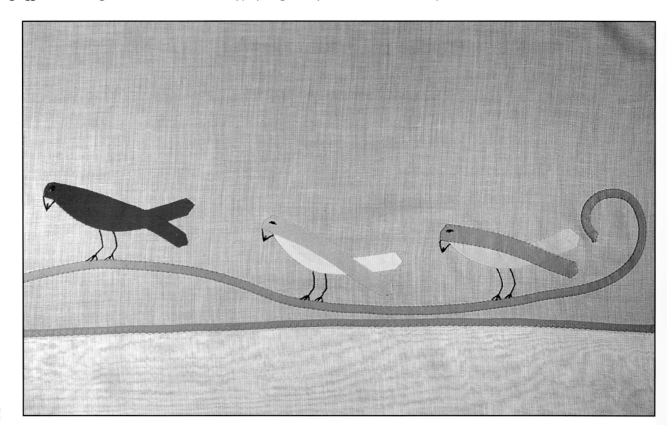

Handkerchief Aprons

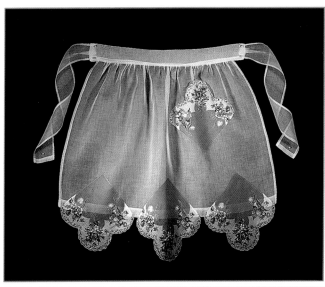

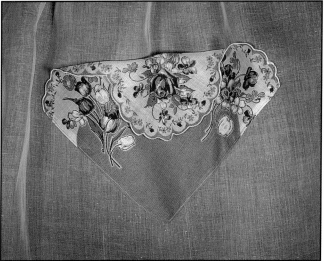

A lavender handkerchief with scalloped edging and bouquets of red roses and tulips has been cut into **four equal parts** for this sunny yellow gathered organdy apron. Three quarters are machine-stitched on point at the bottom. The fourth quarter is inverted for a frilly pocket with fold down top.

While one may consider the handkerchief a mostly functional item, the handkerchief *apron* clearly falls into the decorative category. Hanky aprons are lightweight, sometimes even flimsy, and pretty to look at. They are among the most beautiful aprons. This is so because the maker probably selected her loveliest or favorite handkerchiefs to incorporate into the design.

Handkerchief aprons consist largely of two main styles—those composed of handkerchief fabric *only* and those made from a combination of a handkerchief (or handkerchiefs) and another lightweight fabric, usually a sheer batiste, lawn, or organdy. The latter style seems to be more common.

The collection of handkerchief aprons featured here includes colorful floral bouquets in rosy pinks, regal purple, sparkling yellow, autumn gold, lustrous lavenders, and soft greens—each a feast for the eyes.

The 'handkerchief only' apron requires three identical handkerchiefs, which comprise the entire body of the apron. One hanky is used intact for the main front panel of the apron. A second hanky is cut diagonally into halves for the sides of the apron. A third hanky is cut lengthwise into halves for the lower front portion.

This classic 'three-hanky' apron usually has a grosgrain (or less commonly, satin) ribbon for the combination waistband and sashes. Fullness is created at the center bottom with several pleats or gathers, or more rarely, a flared cut. It rarely has pockets.

The other more common style—a combination of one handkerchief with lightweight fabric—can be crafted in several ways. Following are four methods to prepare a hanky for design application:

1. Cut into quarter sections, horizontally and vertically
2. Cut into quarter sections, diagonally
3. Cut into halves, diagonally
4. Uncut (hanky remains intact)

Examples of all four preparation methods as they have been made into aprons are included.

What you *won't* find in this section are remnants and recycled fabrics. All the aprons are assembled from new fabrics and new handkerchiefs. What you *will* find are beautifully designed handkerchiefs and cleverly crafted aprons.

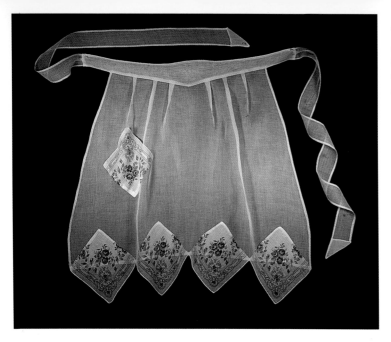

You'll need **more than one handkerchief** to make this design. Five quarter sections are required—four for the lower border, and one for the pocket. All pieces are machine-stitched to the pale yellow organdy. The attractively shaped waistband is attached with six opposing half-inch pleats.

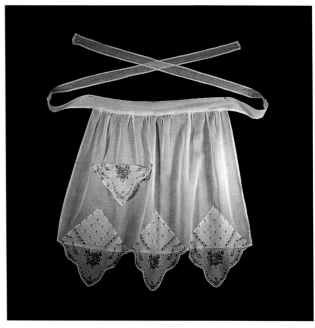

A handkerchief with a bordered edge and **yellow hearts and purple flowers** corner motif has been similarly quartered and stitched on point for this gathered apron. The pocket is placed at the right and the white fabric is soft cotton lawn. The handkerchief has a hand-rolled hem.

Mint green organdy is the background choice for this handkerchief of golden roses and blue forget-me-nots. Application of metallic gold rickrack in sharp V's and across the pocket top makes for **a glitzy arrangement**. The pocket quarter has been angled at the sides, folded at the top, and trimmed with golden rickrack.

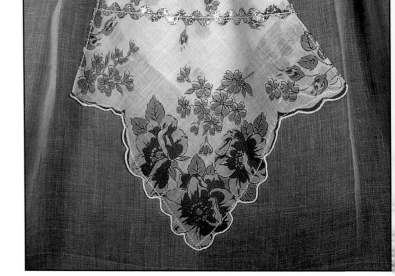

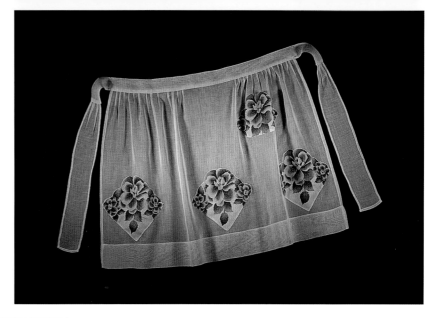

Breathtaking blooms in purple and lavender are set on point and appliquéd in free-floating sections on this snowy white batiste apron. The generously wide skirt is finely pleated at the waist. The pocket has been artfully shaped and stitched, leaving a side-only entry.

Take **a beautiful flowered handkerchief.** Cut it diagonally into two parts. Place them with the long sides at the top edge of a widely-hemmed pleated organdy apron. Appliqué in place. These hanky sections are ever so slightly overlapped at the center.

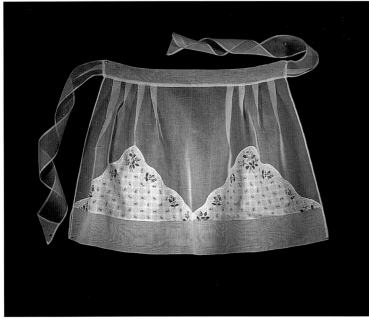

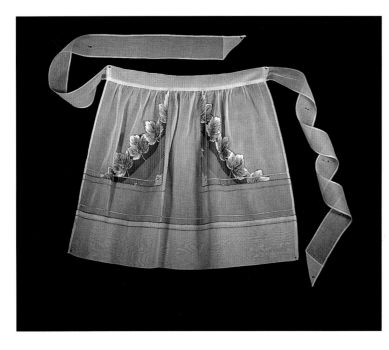

Take another large colorful handkerchief (A maple leaf design will do nicely.). Cut it diagonally into four parts. Set two parts aside (for another apron?). Place the remaining parts at 90-degree angles to create **a twin-pocketed symmetrical arrangement.** Trim with three shades of miniature golden rickrack.

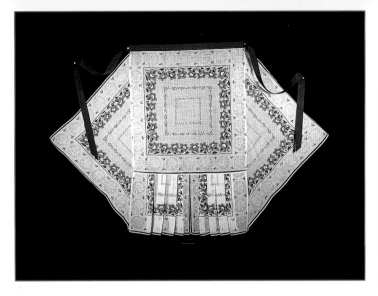

One square, two triangles, and two rectangles make a three-hanky apron. Garlands of delicate five-petaled flowers form the borders of these hankies. A 5/8-inch wide navy blue grosgrain ribbon is used for the combination waistband/sash.

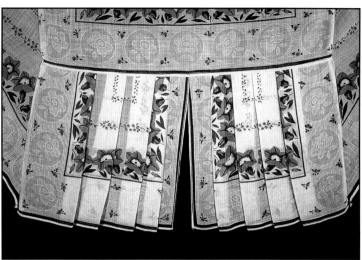

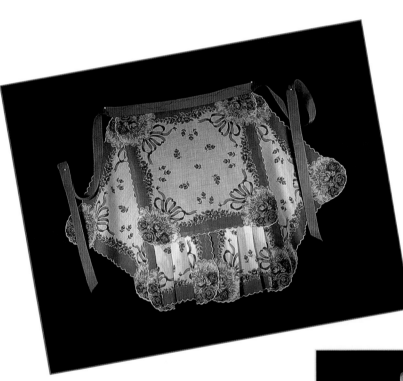

Three hankies with **bouquets of red roses** and flowing ribbons at each corner make this among the showiest of handkerchief aprons. The lower center section has a center vent and three deep pleats at each side. A bizarre orange grosgrain ribbon tops the apron.

Sunny yellow and lilac (complementary colors on the color wheel) combine in this pleasant three-hanky apron of dainty floral sprays. Barely detectable scalloped edges fringe each hanky. **Precisely pleated** at the lower edge (twelve half-inch pleats), the apron is topped with yellow grosgrain ribbon.

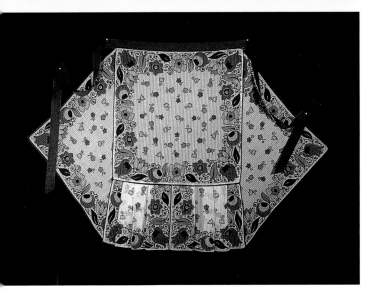

Orange and golden flowers on a striped background lend **an autumnal feeling** to this apron. The handkerchiefs also include a touch of turquoise and a dose of brown for foliage. A one-inch-wide deep forest green grosgrain waistband/sash completes the design. The six-pleated section is stitched shut at the bottom center.

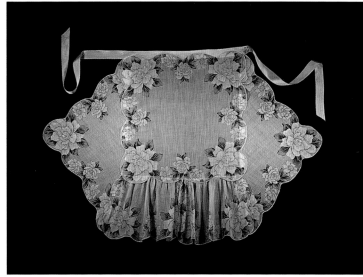

Shiny **pink satin ribbon sashes** and huge showy white roses set this handkerchief apron apart from the others. In typical three-hanky fashion, one has been cut diagonally, one horizontally, and one left intact. The gently scalloped edges and pale pink background lend to this simply elegant design. The lower center pieces have been overlapped and stitched shut.

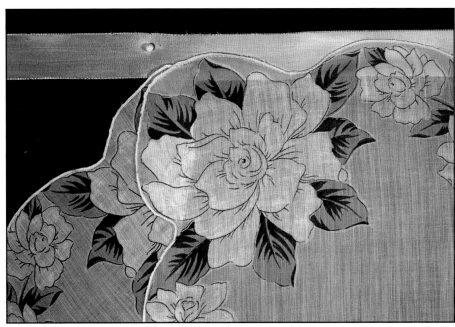

The conventional three-handkerchief apron has been modified in two ways on this design. **Two angled pockets** are attached to the side triangles, and bright yellow and gold metallic rickrack is used to trim the outer edges and pockets. Four hankies are required for this apron, which is topped with a one-piece combination waistband/sash of translucent white organdy.

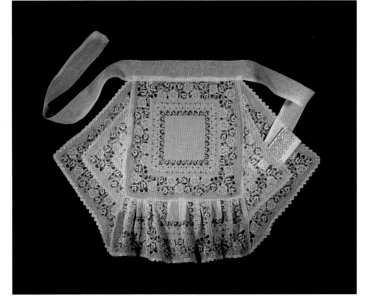

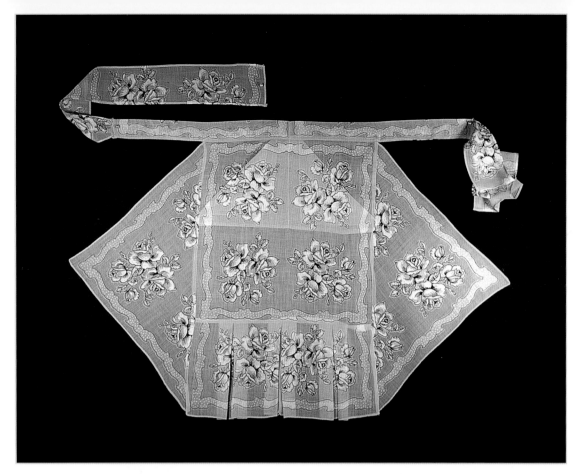

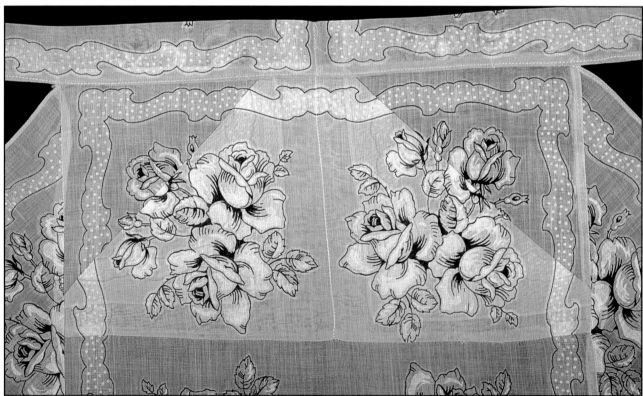

Yet another unique pocket style can be found on this handkerchief apron. An additional hanky is needed for the two angled pockets, which have been cleverly placed at the center top. Care has been taken to accurately match the floral designs and white flowing borders on each hanky. Excess pieces have been used to design the pieced and extended waistband and sashes. From the collection of Betty Wilson.
Check The Color Purple section for two more handkerchief style aprons.

Pockets for Every Purpose

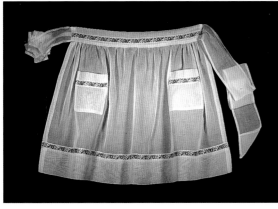

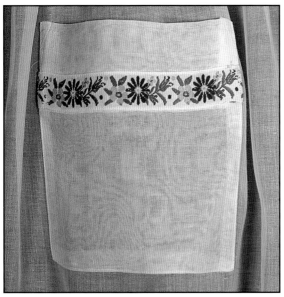

This immaculate white organdy gathered apron features pockets in their most common arrangement: **squared, paired, and decorated**. Floral trim in bright red, yellow, blue, and green adds just the right touch of beauty. All trim is machine-stitched, and the pockets are top-stitched and reinforced at the upper corners.

Many apron wearers would agree that the most important part of an apron is the pocket. And more than one is better. Of course, some aprons do not have a pocket. This would surely be considered a serious oversight by those who view aprons as primarily functional. One pocket is essential. Two are even better. And three pockets are an unusual extravagance.

One pocket seems to be the norm. In any given selection of aprons you will find everything from no pockets to numerous pockets, one or two being most common. Additional pockets are found on the more practical styles, few or none on the purely decorative styles. The winner of the "apron with the most pockets" (eight little compartments) is pictured in this section.

The assortment of pocket styles is vast. If you thought there were only two kinds of pockets—rounded at the bottom or squared at the bottom, you're in for a surprise. More than thirty-five different styles are found throughout the book. Innovative shapes and clever placements abound. There are few opportunities for novel design on an apron. The pocket is an ideal place for the designer or maker to display a fresh idea.

The variety of apron pocket treatments is impressive. When contrasted with the pocket styles used on men's shirts, there is simply no comparison. A man's shirt pocket is a fairly generic thing—square, perhaps with a flap or mock flap, perhaps a button. You see one, you've seen 'em all. Not so in the world of apron pockets. Variety and novelty run rampant.

In addition to the number and shape of apron pockets, we can consider the location, attachment method, direction of entry, and embellishments. Pocket location may seem obvious—on the right side (if you're right-handed), just a few inches below the waistband. This appears to be the most conventional, if not the most convenient place. And that's where most of them are located. But you'll also find them in a number of other surprising places, some so secret that they cannot be detected visually. In addition to the obvious right, left, and even center front locations, look for pockets on waistbands, in seams, on side panels, at the bottom edge, and even on the inside of the apron. Some are so well inserted or camouflaged they defy detection.

Techniques for attachment include appliqué (the commonly referred-to "patch" pocket), side insertion, seam insertion, waistband insertion, attachment to the bottom, or any combination of these methods. By far, the most common method is application on the skirt panel. Insertion in a seam is less frequent. Clever designers have even placed pockets in separate side panels.

Secret or camouflaged pockets are among the more fascinating designs. Pockets may be incorporated into overlapping panel sections, hidden inside the waistband, or placed with precisely matched fabric and color.

The tiniest pockets are located on the waistband and measure only 2 1/4 inches deep and 3 1/2 inches wide—less than eight square inches. Their intent is perhaps purely decorative, but they could be used for small objects such as a key, a ring, or a neatly folded facial tissue. In contrast, the largest pocket measures 13 inches deep and 34 inches wide—more than two square feet! This 'mother of all pockets' is obviously a storage or gathering type, designed for carrying larger quantities or numerous items, e.g., vegetables from the garden, clothespins for the laundry, supplies for whatever task is at hand, personal items, or maybe even a snack or lunch.

One logically assumes the pocket entry is from the top. In fact, many pockets have side, center front, or even angled entries. A few have dual entries. Of the many pocket styles examined, the overwhelming majority were top entry. The remaining pockets were about equally divided among side entry, center front entry, angled entry, and dual entry.

What about the size of a pocket? How does one measure it? By depth? By width? In inches? By whether or not you can fit your hand into it? Or your entire hand plus additional objects? One method of describing the size of a pocket is by the number of fingers of a flattened hand you can insert into it. This applies, of course, to little pockets, i.e., those smaller than your hand. A five-finger pocket is one into which you can just barely slip all five fingers. A four-finger pocket will accommodate four fingers. A three-finger pocket is slightly smaller. A two-finger pocket is so tiny its practicality might be questioned (unless it's on a child's apron).

Finally, observations can be made about pocket embellishments. Embroidery, rickrack, ruffles, lace, bows, binding, pleating, and smocking have all been used for decoration. With such adornments, the pocket becomes the focal point. No longer merely a functional space, it now commands our visual attention.

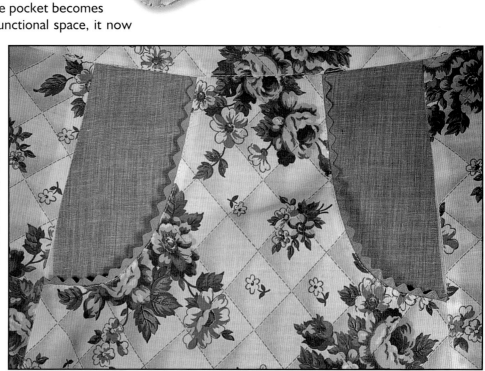

The main distinction of this organdy and percale apron is the **dual-entry center pocket,** a prime example of the blending of function and decoration. Other design features include an ever so slightly shaped waist and a lower gathered inset. The lovely floral bouquets are complemented by honey gold rickrack trim.

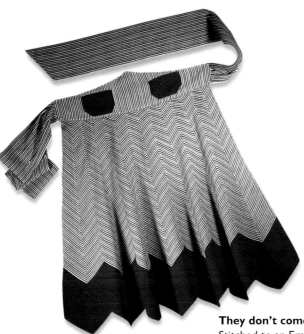

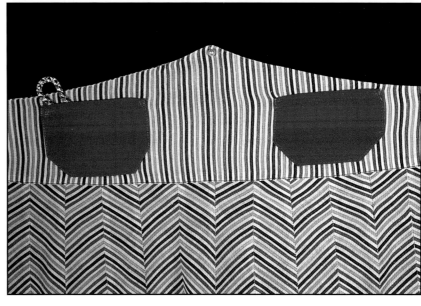

They don't come much smaller than this—each red pocket measures 2 1/4 by 3 1/2 inches. Stitched to an Empire waistband and set atop a 14-gore apron, perhaps they could hold a ring, a key, or other small item. Or maybe they're purely decorative. Have you ever seen so many meticulously matched stripes?

Surely you will have storage space to spare in this huge **mother of all pockets.** It measures 34 inches wide and is 13 inches at its deepest point. It has been strategically tacked at the lower inner corners, in effect making four interconnected compartments. White rickrack edges the pocket and tops the five-inch deep hem.

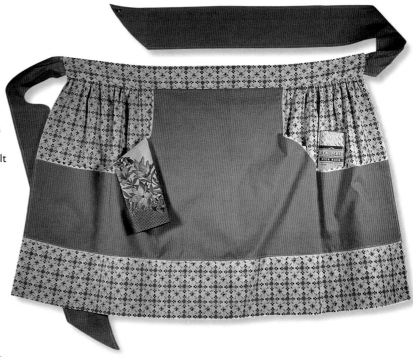

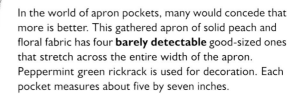

In the world of apron pockets, many would concede that more is better. This gathered apron of solid peach and floral fabric has four **barely detectable** good-sized ones that stretch across the entire width of the apron. Peppermint green rickrack is used for decoration. Each pocket measures about five by seven inches.

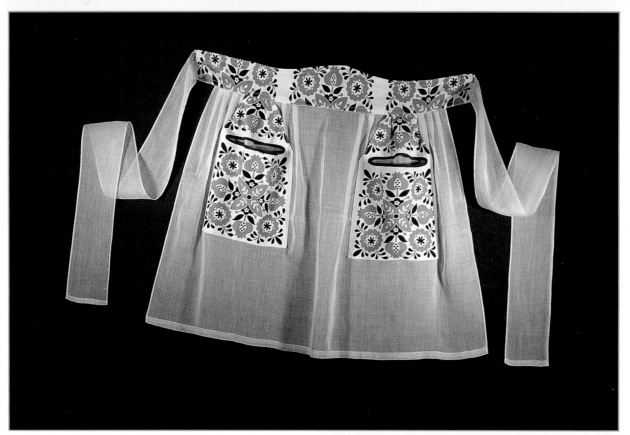

Two kelly-green and black **front entry pockets** grace this white organdy apron. Carefully placed graphic floral designs highlight the pockets, which are appliquéd to the skirt front and pleated at the waistline. Pocket openings are finished with black bias tape. The shaped waistband and pockets are carefully top-stitched in white.

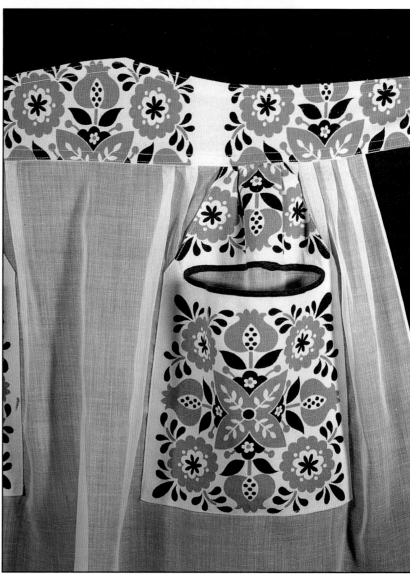

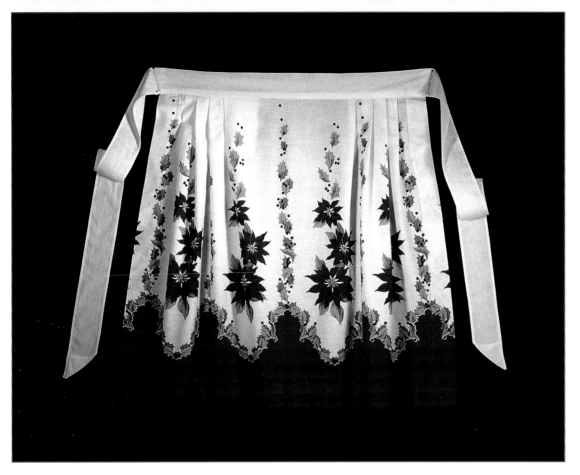

This vibrant border printed holly berry and poinsettia apron is sure to instill the holiday spirit. Details include red top stitching, mitered corners in the hem, and eight waistline pleats. What the guests won't detect is the **secret pocket** appliquéd to the inside of the waistband. At more than twenty-four inches from top to bottom, this apron is one of the longest.

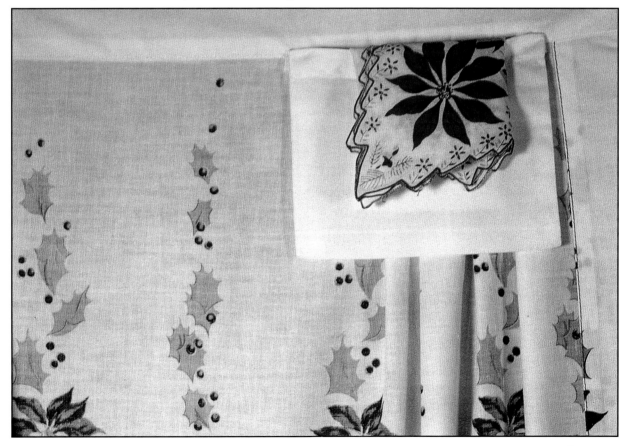

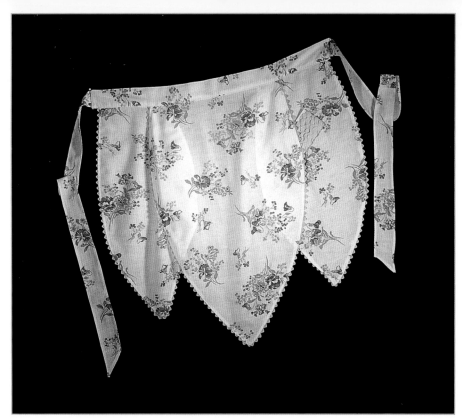

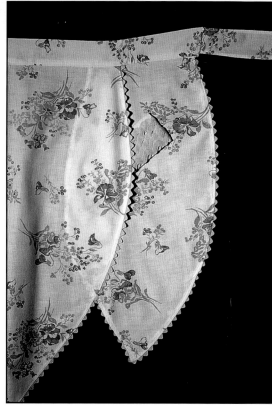

Two **not-so-obvious** elongated pockets with convex outer edges are created by the overlapping of the three sections in this apron. The pockets are well-hidden, detectable only by the machine stitching and rickrack edging. The large pink and blue floral bouquets are complemented with pink rickrack trim. Can you tell that this apron is made from a recycled cotton bag?

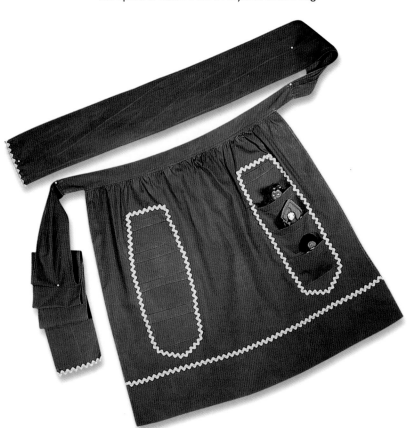

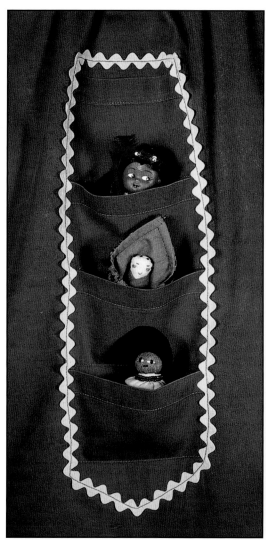

Winning honors for **the apron with the most pockets** is this chocolate brown cotton gathered design. Eight tiny banded pockets are stacked and stitched to the skirt. Yellow rickrack outlines each panel of pockets and the lower edge of this wide-hemmed, wide-sashed apron. Each pocket measures about 2 1/2 by 4 inches; each panel about 4 by 12 inches.

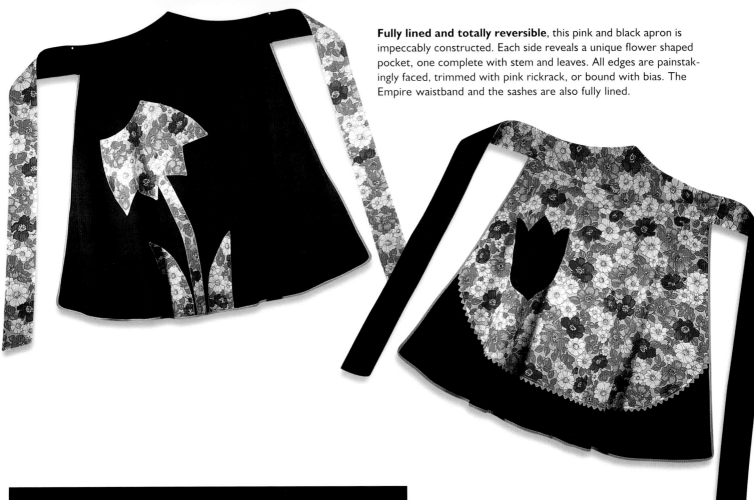

Fully lined and totally reversible, this pink and black apron is impeccably constructed. Each side reveals a unique flower shaped pocket, one complete with stem and leaves. All edges are painstakingly faced, trimmed with pink rickrack, or bound with bias. The Empire waistband and the sashes are also fully lined.

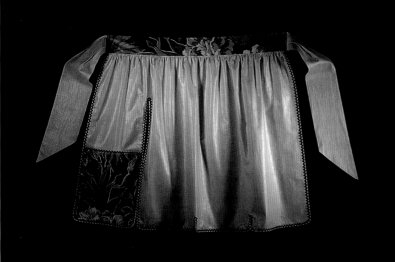

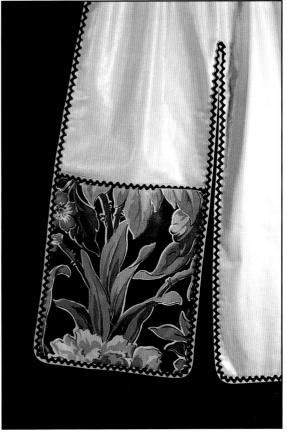

You'll need to reach to the right for this **side panel pocket**. Separated by a deep slit, this exotic flowered fabric is a fine complement to the buttery yellow polished cotton. Miniature black rickrack is used to outline the pocket panel and apron edges. The lower edge is accented with one-inch notches.

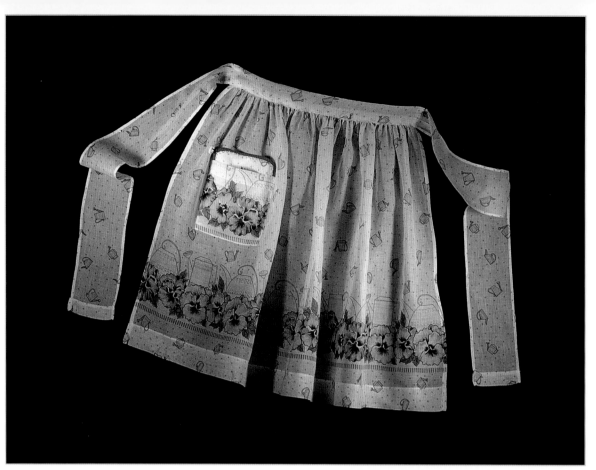

A garden theme with sprinkling cans and a border of pansies dominates this gathered organdy apron. The pansy motif is repeated in the pocket. What's so special is not the pocket itself, but **what's in it**—a potholder made from the same fabric as the apron. The perimeter of the potholder is feather-stitched with shiny gold embroidery floss.

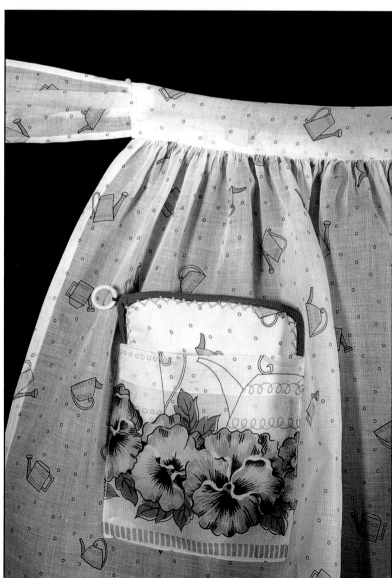

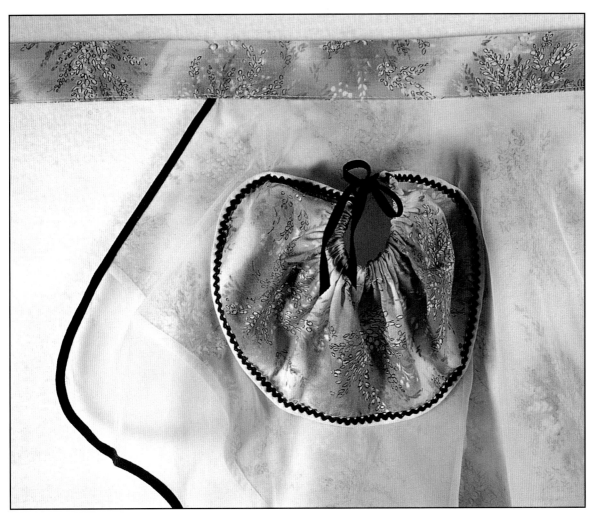

You'll need to use two settings on your iron when you press this flared and floral apron of sheer nylon and cotton calico. Cool for nylon, hot for cotton. Other unusual features include the reversible overskirting and the **fancy draw-string pockets**, each highlighted with minia-ture black rickrack and black bias drawstrings.

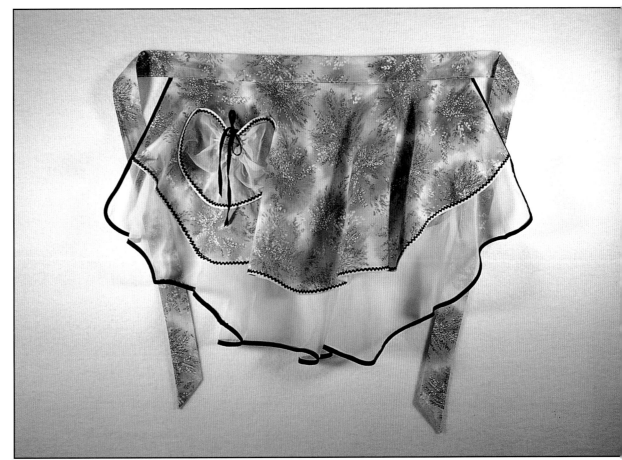

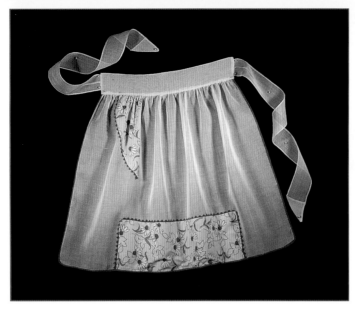

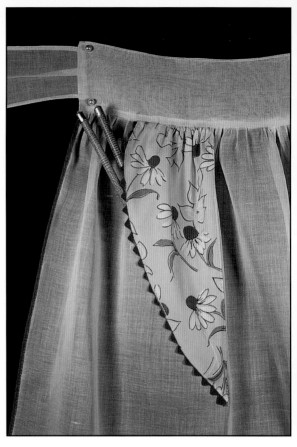

Tall and slender might be two words to describe this odd-shaped pocket. Bright pink rickrack and bias trim outline the sides of the pocket, the lower panel, and the outer edges. Cotton organdy forms the main body of this gathered apron, and a 1950s-style daisy floral fabric in lime green brings it to life.

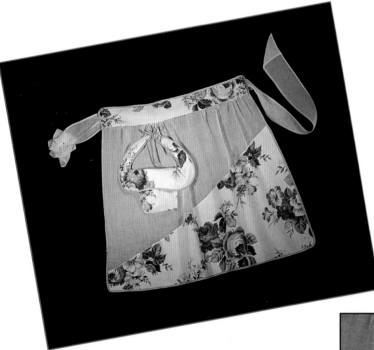

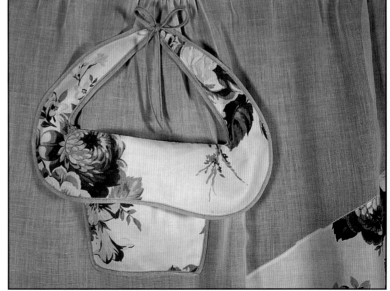

An unusual rounded collar tops the pocket of this organdy and percale apron. The pocket is edged with light green bias trim, which forms a bow at the apex of the pocket extension. Colorful and showy floral arrangements and a sweeping diagonal line add further elegance to this dressy serving apron.

Section Three

COLOR GALLERY

Seeing Red

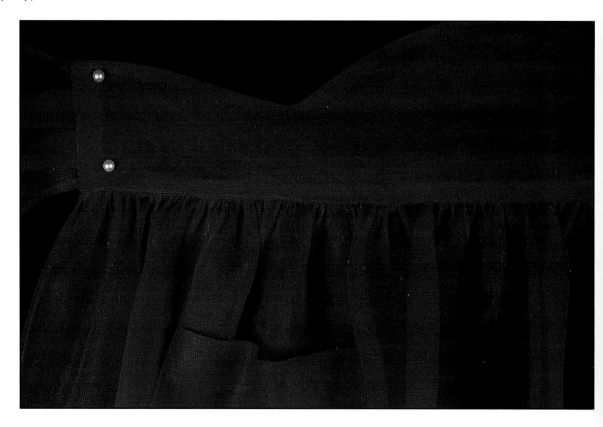

Four color groupings have been selected for the Gallery: Red, pink, yellow, and purple. The choice of these four and the elimination of other color categories was rather arbitrary. All the primary and secondary hues in the traditional color wheel (red, yellow, blue, orange, green, purple) were considered. As were the seven colors of the spectrum (red, orange, yellow, green, blue, indigo, violet). Also, thought was given to the fifteen colors of the gingham aprons in the *Every Color Under the Sun* section. But restrictions had to be made. Here are some reasons for inclusion of these four groups:

1. **Red** is very graphic visually, and red aprons are abundant.
2. **Pink** aprons are also prevalent, and pink most definitely and clearly conveys traditional femininity.
3. I like **yellow**.
4. **Purple** is the opposite of yellow on the color wheel, and I also like *it* (in aprons, anyway).

This dramatic scarlet organdy apron is sure to brighten the dining room and capture the attention of guests. Three gentle curves dominate the lower edge of the apron, the bottom of the pocket, and the shaped and gathered waistband. **Deep and wide** are the words that clearly describe the six-inch hem and the five-and-a-half-inch sashes, which are attached with two generous pleats. The sash ends are cleverly cut into curves that resemble a 'whale's tail'.

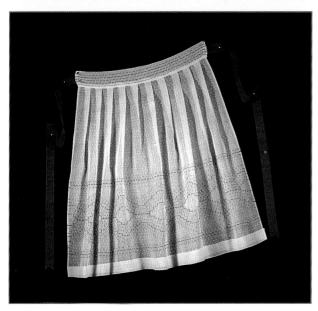

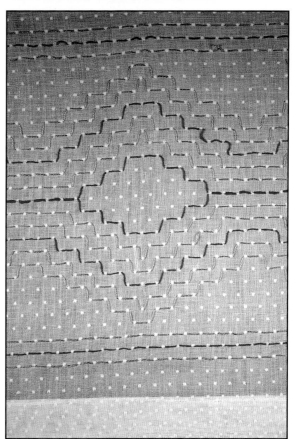

Elongated, loosely connected **red and green running stitches** are used in this expansive (eight inches wide) stair step border design. Widely spaced flocked dots on cotton organdy serve as the guidelines for stitching. Five rows of stitches decorate the waistband, and grosgrain ribbon sashes have been added to this one-way pleated apron.

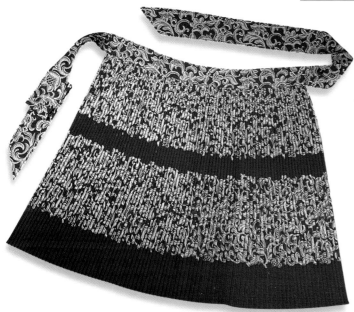

Surely **the ultimate in pleating**, this red, white, and gray apron packs 90 accordion-style pleats into a 17-inch span. That makes each pleat about 3/16 inch. It was called the 'sweet pleat' Glam-o-Apron (as advertised in *Life*!). Found in its original packaging, this apron has never been worn.

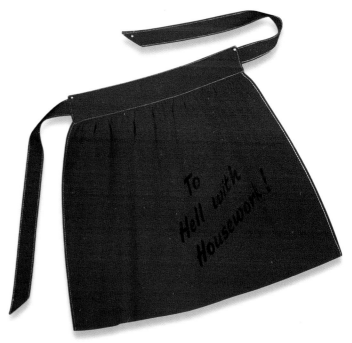

One of the rare "documentary aprons," this **"To Hell with Housework"** design is certain to stimulate (or stifle?) conversation. Lightly gathered and top-stitched in extra large white machine stitches, this blood-red muslin apron is clearly one with attitude. What? No pocket? Guess you won't need one if you're not doing housework.

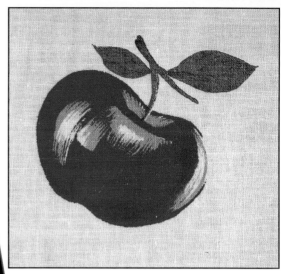

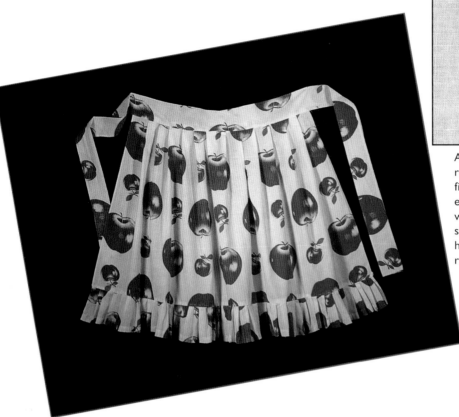

Among the cheeriest and brightest of fabrics, this red apple apron is **entirely hand-sewn**, including fine hemming stitches up and down the length of each sash. Deep waistline pleats and a lower ruffle with uneven pleats accent this well used and slightly stained cotton apron. Notice the lingering hand-basted stitches at the upper edge of the ruffle.

A **stylized stag and floral fabric** is the main attraction in this lightweight cotton organdy apron. The U-shaped twin pockets and perimeter are edged with a combination rickrack and ruffle trim. The upper edge of this pear-shaped design is ever-so-slightly gathered.

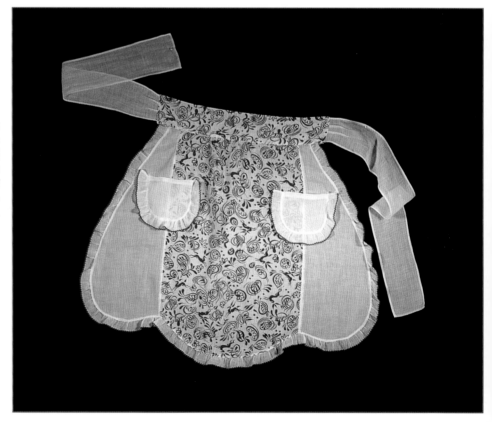

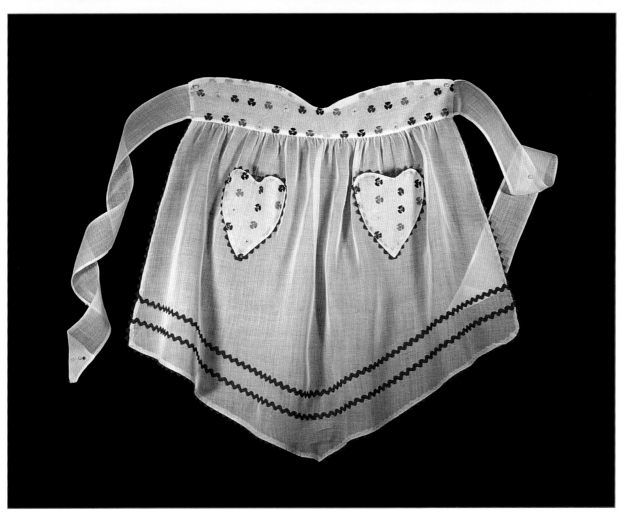

Machine-embroidered flowers in bright red, yellow, blue, and green are the spotlight in this unusually shaped cotton organdy apron. Gentle curves of the two **heart-shaped pockets** are echoed in the upper waistband. Crimson red rickrack trims the lower area, pockets, and perimeter of this especially photogenic design.

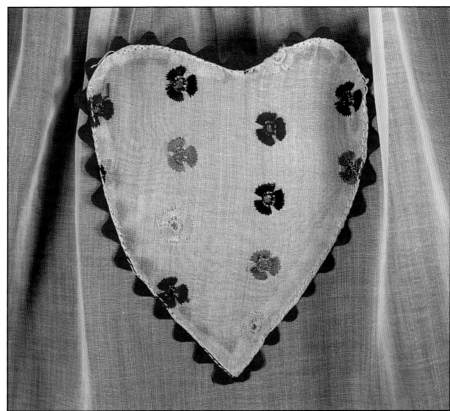

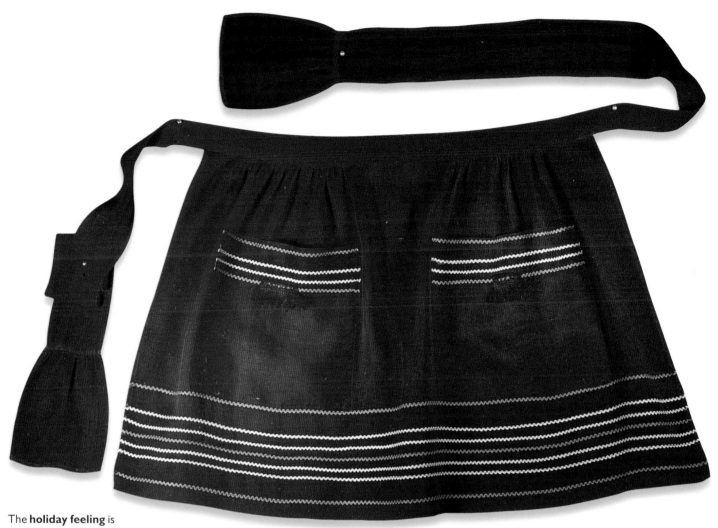

The **holiday feeling** is easily detected in this finely gathered see-through scarlet apron. Narrow rickrack in three colors (pink, light green, and dark green) and small fringes decorate the paired oversize pockets. For the final touch, lightly gathered five-inch-wide extensions have been added to the ends of the sashes.

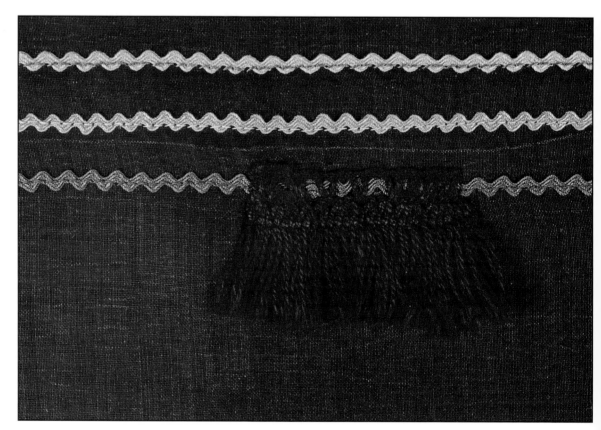

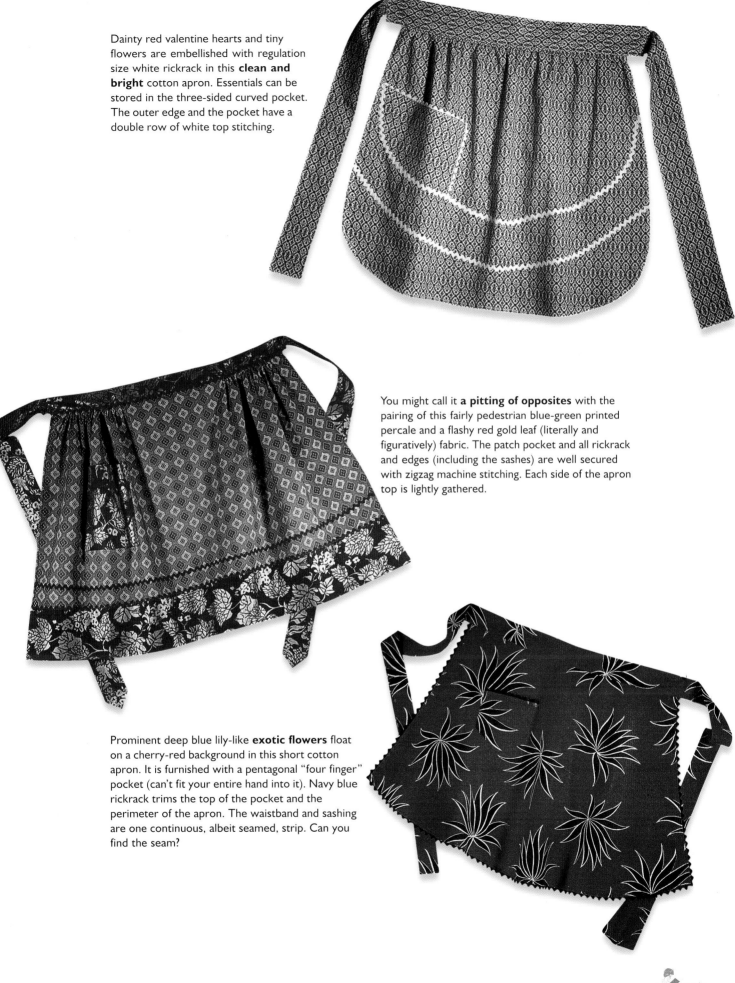

Dainty red valentine hearts and tiny flowers are embellished with regulation size white rickrack in this **clean and bright** cotton apron. Essentials can be stored in the three-sided curved pocket. The outer edge and the pocket have a double row of white top stitching.

You might call it **a pitting of opposites** with the pairing of this fairly pedestrian blue-green printed percale and a flashy red gold leaf (literally and figuratively) fabric. The patch pocket and all rickrack and edges (including the sashes) are well secured with zigzag machine stitching. Each side of the apron top is lightly gathered.

Prominent deep blue lily-like **exotic flowers** float on a cherry-red background in this short cotton apron. It is furnished with a pentagonal "four finger" pocket (can't fit your entire hand into it). Navy blue rickrack trims the top of the pocket and the perimeter of the apron. The waistband and sashing are one continuous, albeit seamed, strip. Can you find the seam?

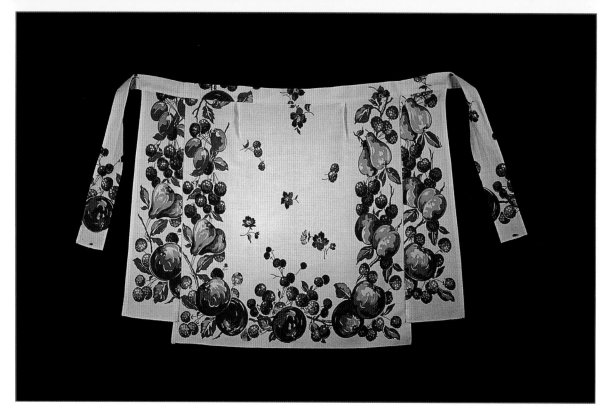

This graphic and very realistic "fruit-of-the-loom" design is a real eye catcher. A cotton towel has been cleverly converted into a modest apron in this colorful print of **peaches, plums, berries, and pears.** One wide central panel and two narrow raised side panels constitute the main portion of the apron. All seams are hand-pieced and the waistband and sashes are hand-hemmed. (The machine stitches at the sides of the apron are hems from the original towel.)

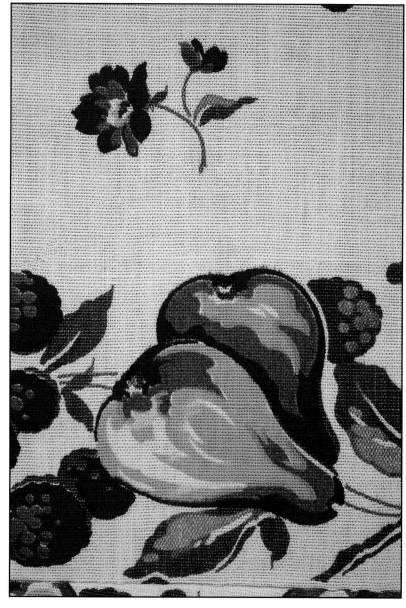

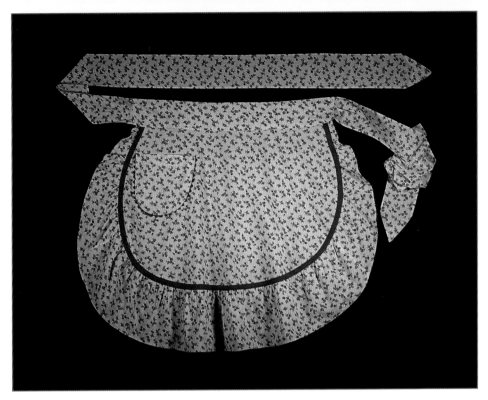

This rounded **calico rose apron** features a graduated semicircular ruffle (from a half inch wide at the top edge to five inches deep at the bottom). It is accented with red bias trim and red rickrack that just barely peaks from behind the outer edge. The U-shaped pocket is likewise edged in rickrack.

Jumbo anthurium flowers and foliage dominate this all cotton apron. A mixture of deep dark reds and olive green on a creamy background lend **a tropical flavor**. The upper edge is secured in multiple miniature pleats. Note the two pocket styles—one large and square, the other smaller and slightly rounded with tiny pleats at the lower edge.

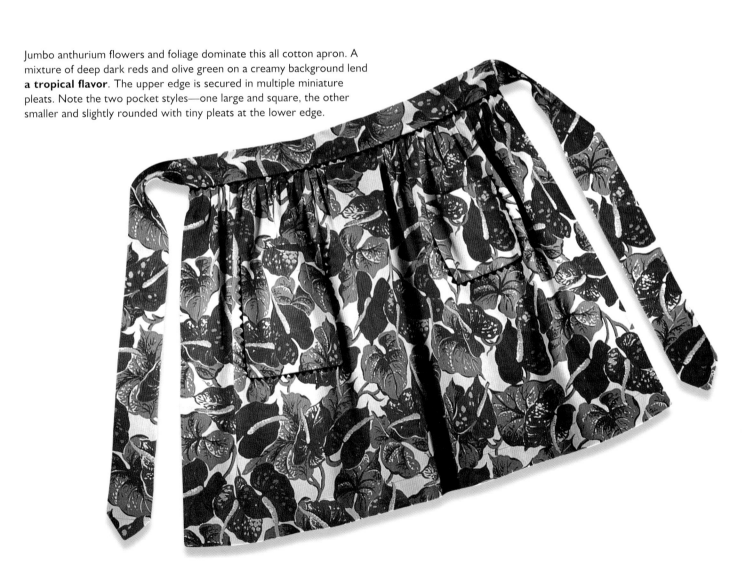

Pretty in Pink

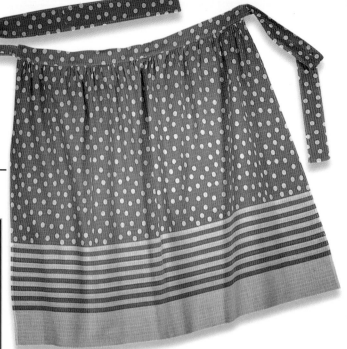

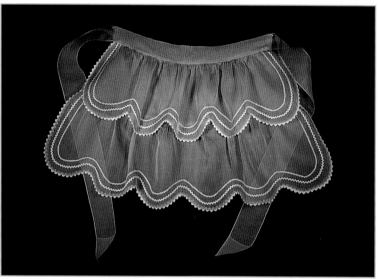

This "**back to the basics**" bubble gum pink apron contrasts white polka dots with pink stripes. It is made from a recycled cotton bag, as evidenced by the tiny holes left from bag stitching and the looser weave of the fabric (lower number of threads per inch). It boasts *no* pocket and *no* hem, the selvage being used at the bottom. Notice that one sash is pieced, due to inadequate fabric length (look for the incomplete white polka dots).

Surely this pink nylon organza apron is the **height of femininity**. The curved and scalloped outer edges and the gathered overskirt lend a ladylike quality to this purely decorative design. It is lavishly trimmed and edged with white rickrack. Note the rickrack in three widths—1/8 inch, 1/4 inch, and 1/2 inch.

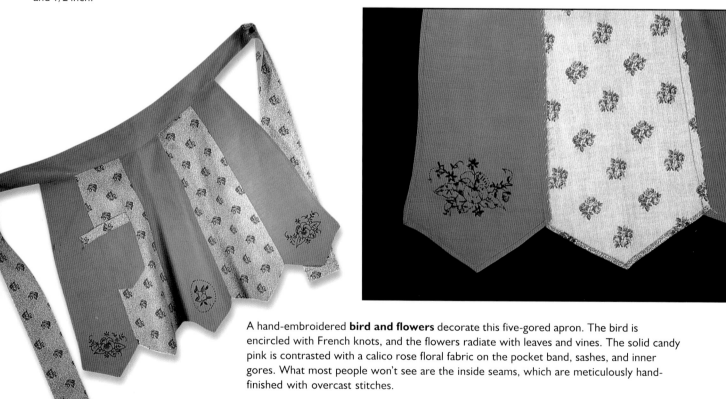

A hand-embroidered **bird and flowers** decorate this five-gored apron. The bird is encircled with French knots, and the flowers radiate with leaves and vines. The solid candy pink is contrasted with a calico rose floral fabric on the pocket band, sashes, and inner gores. What most people won't see are the inside seams, which are meticulously hand-finished with overcast stitches.

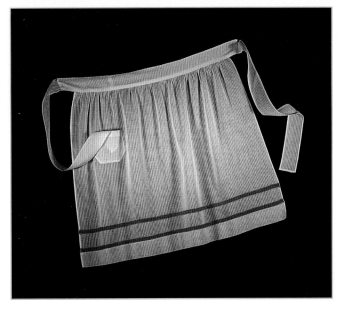

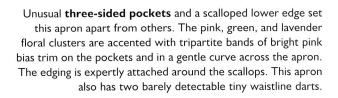

Two horizontal **strips of pink** bias trim accent the lower edge of this apron of gathered lightweight cotton. Notice the narrow stripes and transparency of the frosty white fabric. An unadorned modest hexagonal pocket claims its place on the right. Can you find the seam in the waistband?

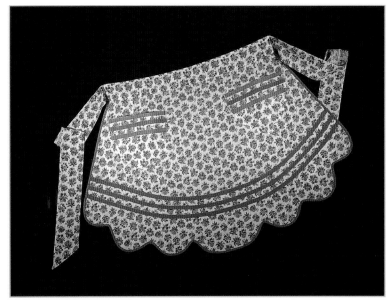

Unusual **three-sided pockets** and a scalloped lower edge set this apron apart from others. The pink, green, and lavender floral clusters are accented with tripartite bands of bright pink bias trim on the pockets and in a gentle curve across the apron. The edging is expertly attached around the scallops. This apron also has two barely detectable tiny waistline darts.

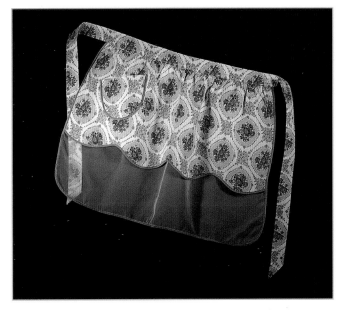

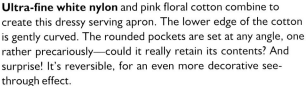

Ultra-fine white nylon and pink floral cotton combine to create this dressy serving apron. The lower edge of the cotton is gently curved. The rounded pockets are set at any angle, one rather precariously—could it really retain its contents? And surprise! It's reversible, for an even more decorative see-through effect.

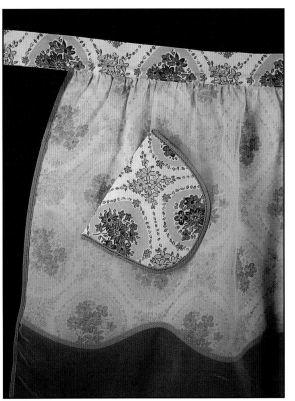

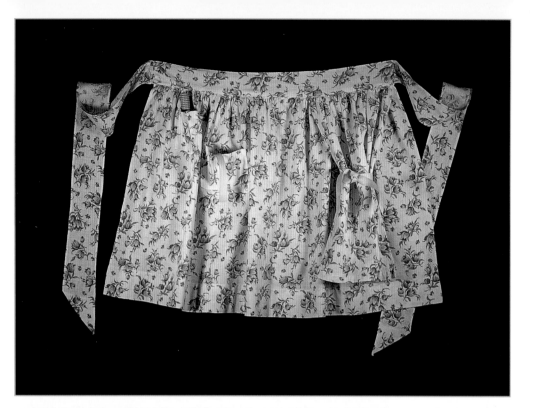

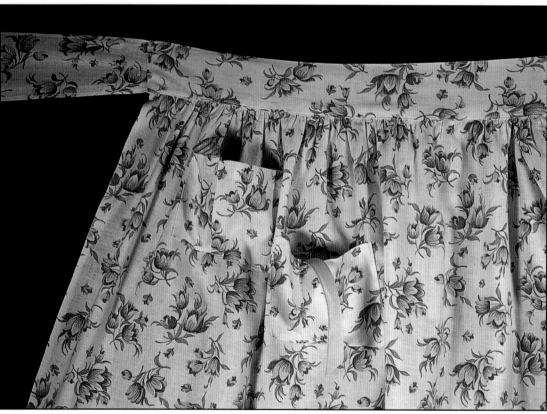

Sensible and functional might be words to describe this pink and green apron, which is made from a recycled cotton bag. The soft and absorbent fabric is gathered at the waistline into a conveniently attached hand towel. Two not-easily-detected rectangular pockets, which are set in stair-step fashion, feature pleats on their lower edges.

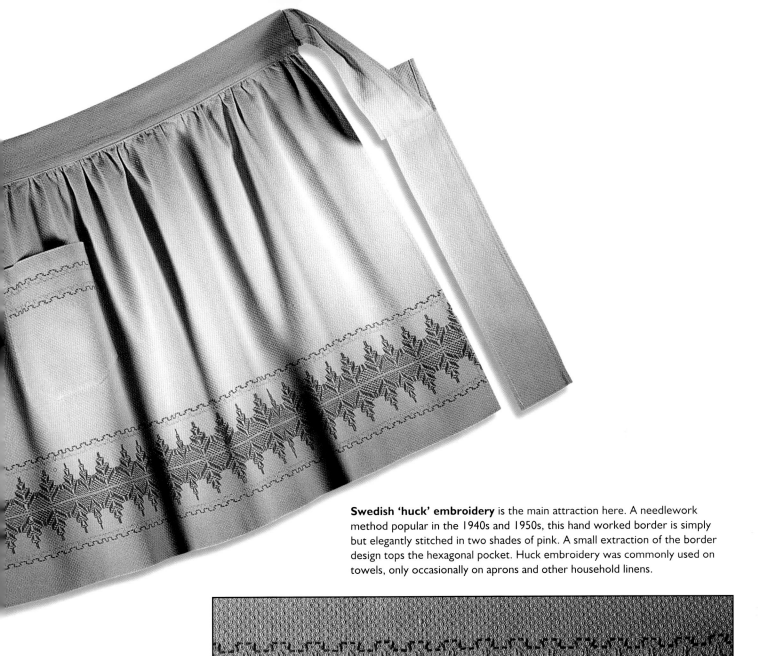

Swedish 'huck' embroidery is the main attraction here. A needlework method popular in the 1940s and 1950s, this hand worked border is simply but elegantly stitched in two shades of pink. A small extraction of the border design tops the hexagonal pocket. Huck embroidery was commonly used on towels, only occasionally on aprons and other household linens.

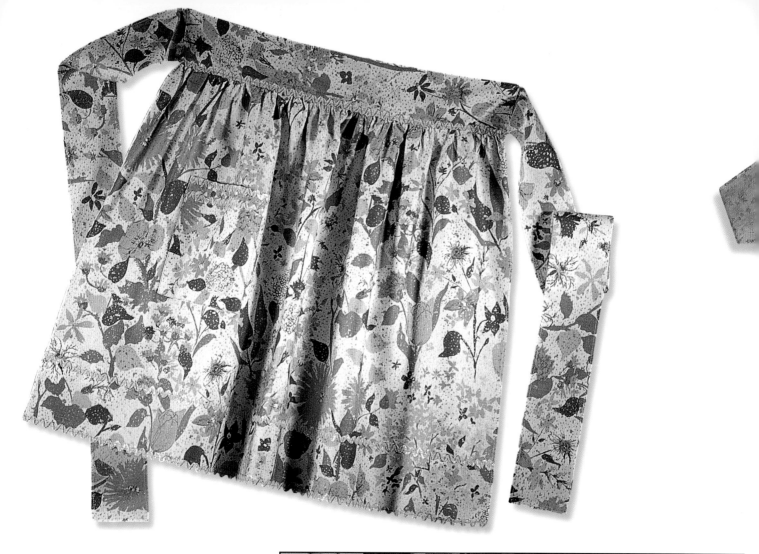

Pink and gold metallic rickrack adds **a little bit of glitz** to this splashy multicolored floral fabric. Parallel strips of trim are top-stitched to the rectangular pocket and along the lower edge. A single row accents the gathered waist.

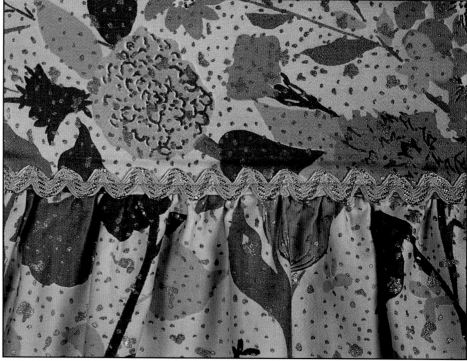

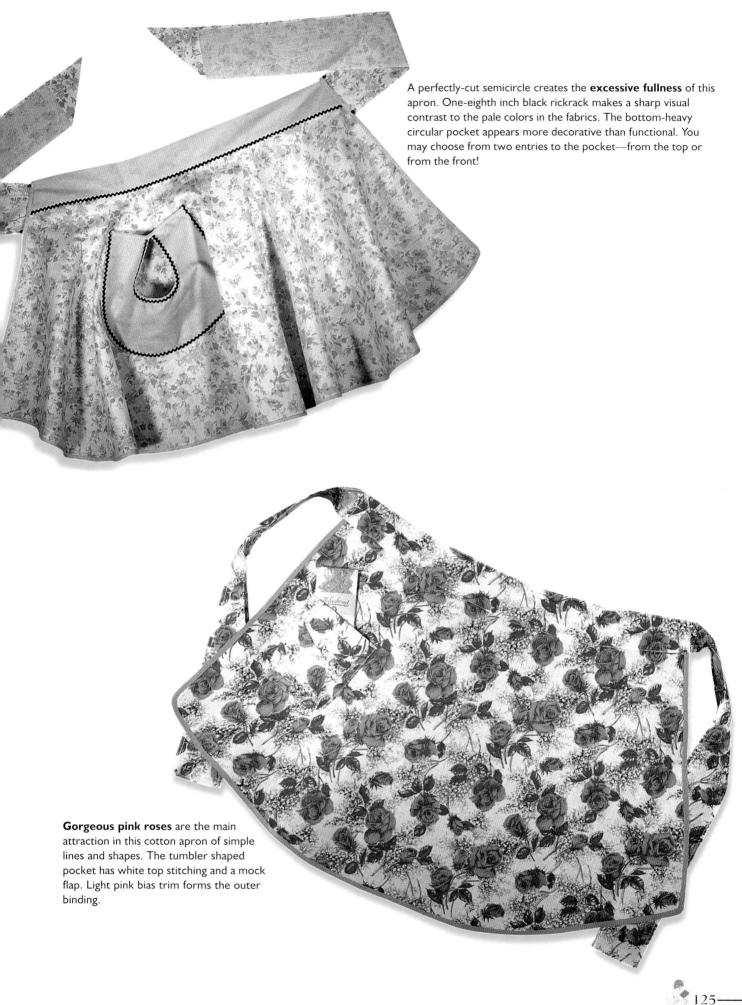

A perfectly-cut semicircle creates the **excessive fullness** of this apron. One-eighth inch black rickrack makes a sharp visual contrast to the pale colors in the fabrics. The bottom-heavy circular pocket appears more decorative than functional. You may choose from two entries to the pocket—from the top or from the front!

Gorgeous pink roses are the main attraction in this cotton apron of simple lines and shapes. The tumbler shaped pocket has white top stitching and a mock flap. Light pink bias trim forms the outer binding.

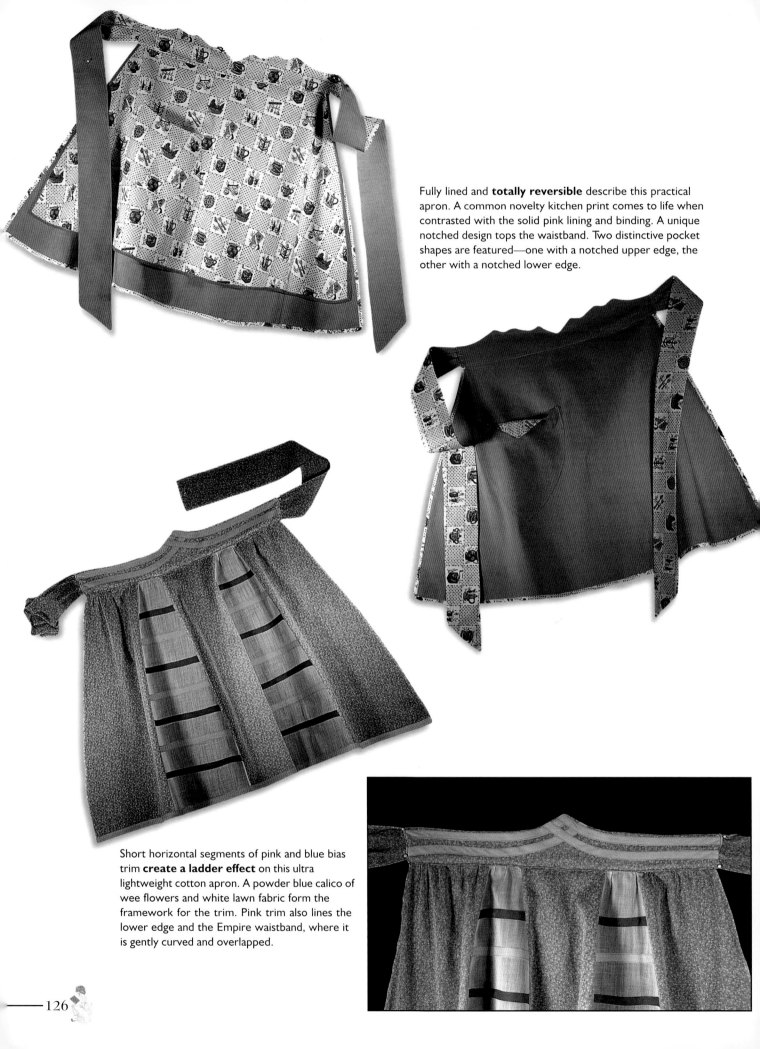

Fully lined and **totally reversible** describe this practical apron. A common novelty kitchen print comes to life when contrasted with the solid pink lining and binding. A unique notched design tops the waistband. Two distinctive pocket shapes are featured—one with a notched upper edge, the other with a notched lower edge.

Short horizontal segments of pink and blue bias trim **create a ladder effect** on this ultra lightweight cotton apron. A powder blue calico of wee flowers and white lawn fabric form the framework for the trim. Pink trim also lines the lower edge and the Empire waistband, where it is gently curved and overlapped.

A Little Bit of Sunshine

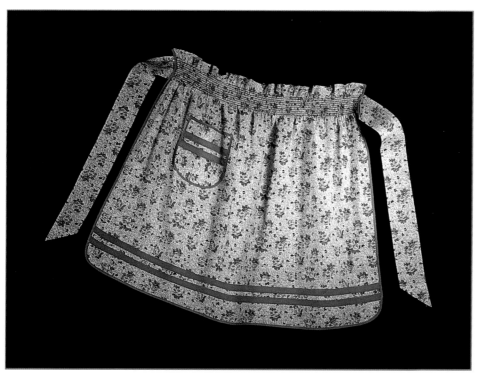

This **sea of yellow roses** is accented with two parallel strips of half-inch green bias trim along the lower edge and on the pocket. The gently rounded apron and pocket edges are also bound in green. The finely pleated and ruffled waistband is the result of ten rows of machine pleating stitches.

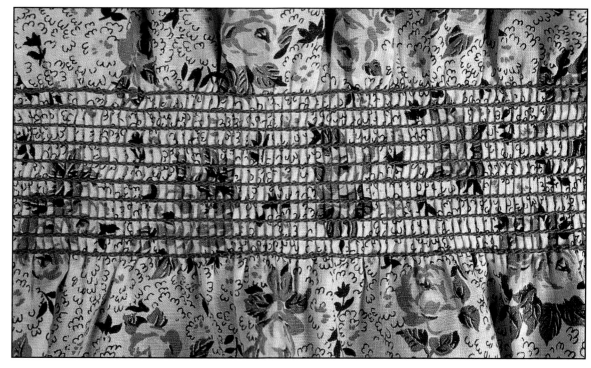

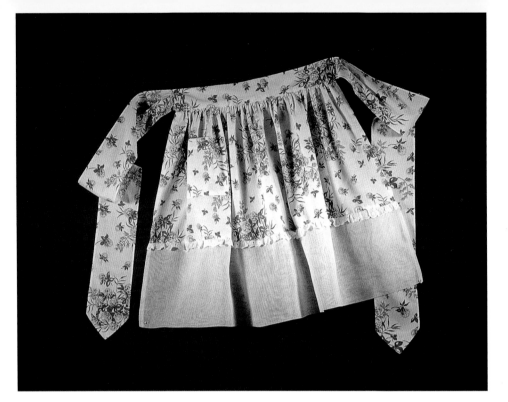

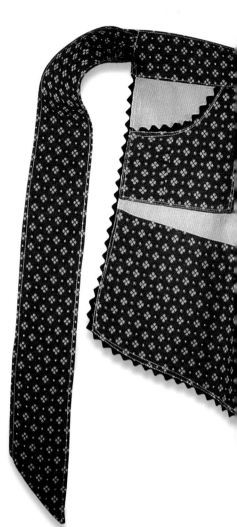

Cotton percale and sheer pale yellow nylon organdy team up in this gathered apron. The **green and lemony yellow floral spray** fabric is edged with 3/4 inch white eyelet lace and a seven-inch lower panel. The extra long and wide sashes are pointed at the ends.

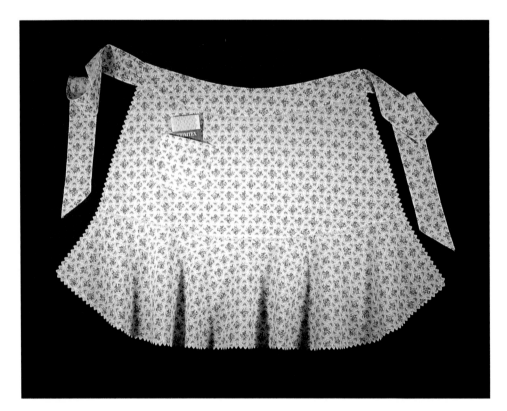

When rickrack was the rage, many calico aprons were trimmed and edged accordingly. This gently curved design is a prime example with its buttery yellow half-inch rickrack trim. The waist is slightly curved and the lower edge is flared. Can you locate the nearly invisible pentagonal patch pocket?

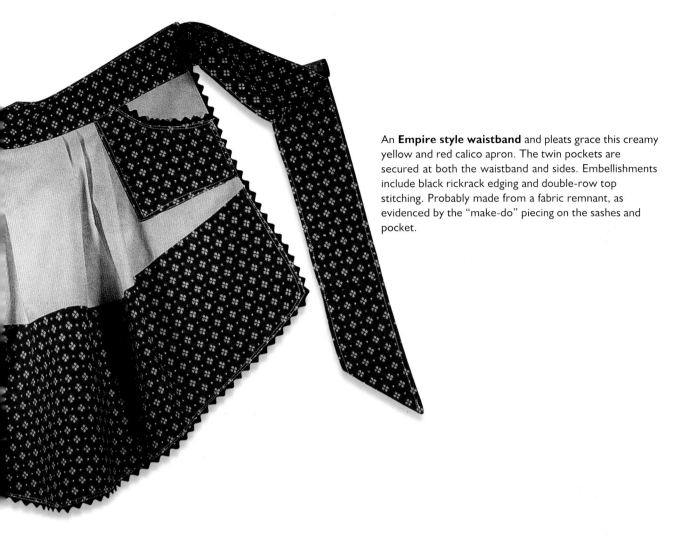

An **Empire style waistband** and pleats grace this creamy yellow and red calico apron. The twin pockets are secured at both the waistband and sides. Embellishments include black rickrack edging and double-row top stitching. Probably made from a fabric remnant, as evidenced by the "make-do" piecing on the sashes and pocket.

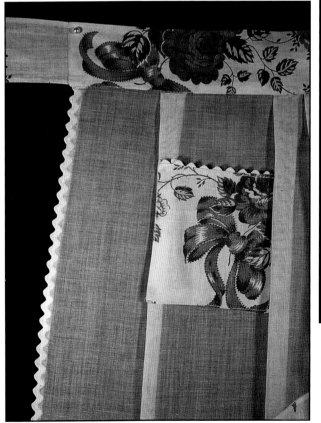

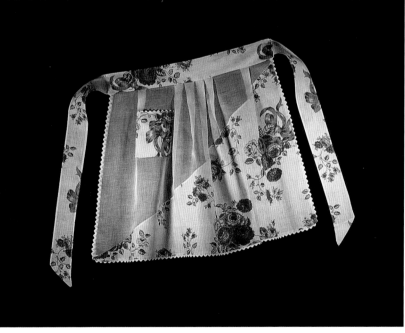

They don't come much prettier than this: A sweeping diagonal line, be-ribboned rose bouquets, and a sunny yellow background. Five one-inch pleats and a patch pocket top the organdy section. White rickrack edging adds the final touch.

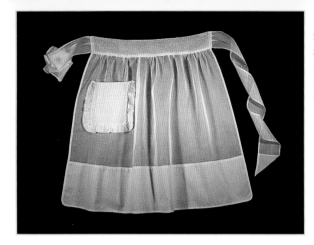

Sheer white organdy and fine yellow checks are the main ingredients of this gathered apron. The squared pocket becomes the focus with its white ruffled edge and bias bound upper edge. Yellow binding outlines the skirt, as well. Notice the **yellow mini rickrack** (about 1/8 inch wide; probably the narrowest available) on the edge of the ruffle.

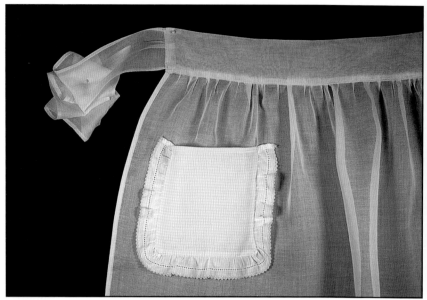

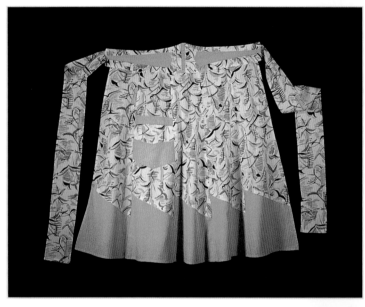

An abstract printed fabric and bright marigold combine in this five gored design. Its maker paid great **attention to detail** with rickrack inserts at the angled lower edges and on the banded pocket. Unusual appliquéd shapes on the Empire style waistband make a statement all their own.

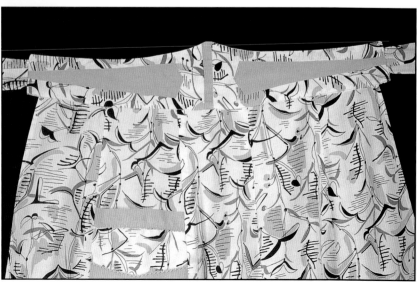

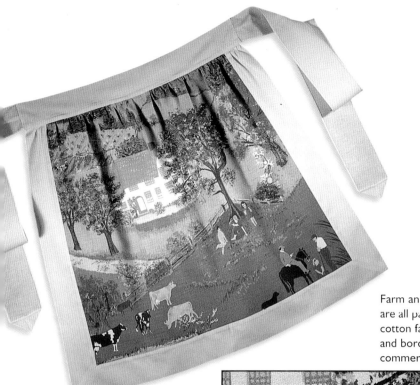

Farm animals, children at play, a country home, trees, and farm fields are all part of **the pastoral scene** on this gathered apron of printed cotton fabric. Solid maize cotton is used for the waistband, sashes, and border, which has mitered corners. This apron carries a commercial label—Maude Tozer, Minneapolis, Minn.

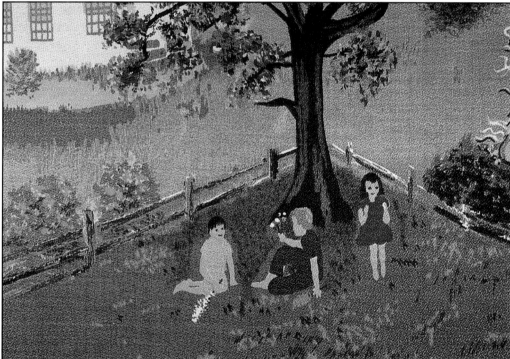

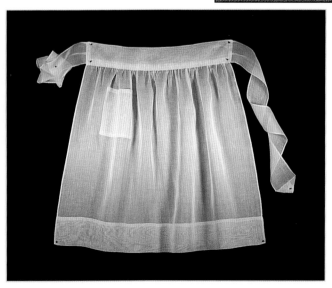

No rickrack, no ruffles, no trim, no lace, no flowers, no checks, no pleats, no embroidery—just **sheer unadorned beauty.**

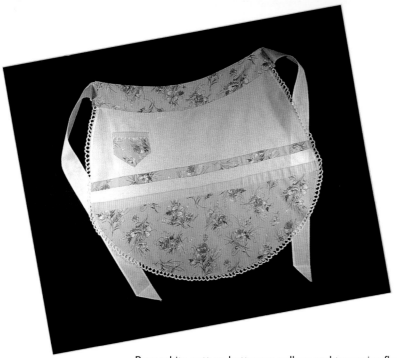

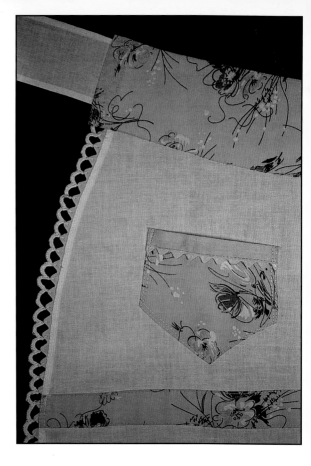

Pure white cotton, buttercup yellow, and turquoise floral fabrics team up in this curved apron. Yellow rickrack and handmade white crochet trim create **a double edged delight.** A shaped waistband and a patch pocket complete this immaculately assembled and stitched design.

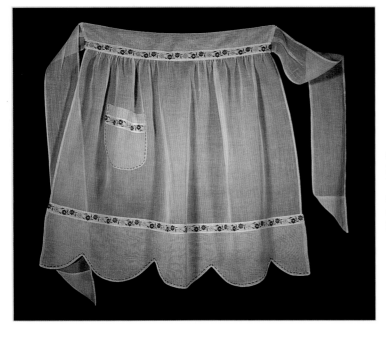

A **scalloped lower edge** that echoes the U-shaped pocket lends drama to this lovely daisy yellow apron. The floral trim with flowers in the three primary colors—red, yellow, and blue—is carefully applied and complemented with decorative running stitches in bright leaf green.

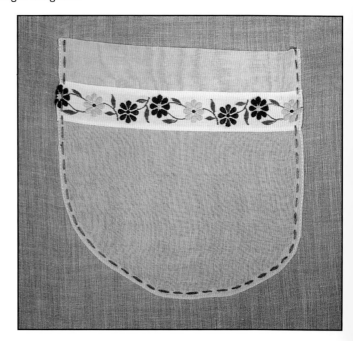

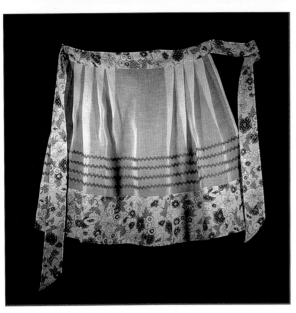

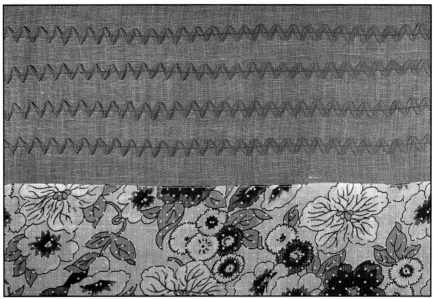

This apron has summertime written all over it. Four parallel rows of kelly green rickrack and a beautiful floral fabric make **the perfect combination** in this deeply pleated design. Crisp translucent white organza forms the backdrop for the lightly flocked and loosely woven red, green, and yellow print. Notice the slightly shaped waistband.

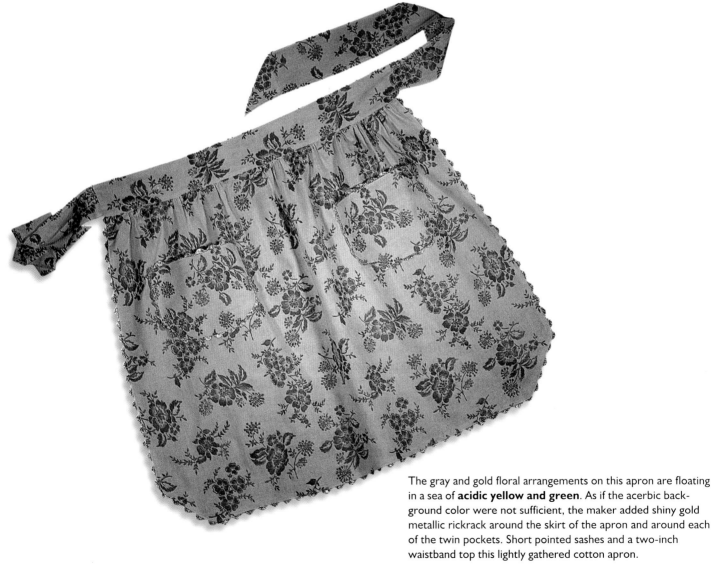

The gray and gold floral arrangements on this apron are floating in a sea of **acidic yellow and green**. As if the acerbic background color were not sufficient, the maker added shiny gold metallic rickrack around the skirt of the apron and around each of the twin pockets. Short pointed sashes and a two-inch waistband top this lightly gathered cotton apron.

The Color Purple
(and Lavender, Lilac, Orchid, and Violet)

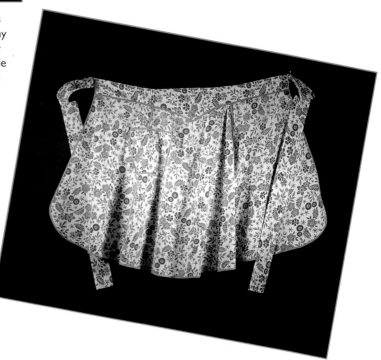

A lavender fine floral cotton and an ash gray solid are used in this **five gore apron**. All seams and edges are carefully bound with pale yellow bias. And (gasp!) there is no pocket. I'm not so certain that the horizontal yellow bias was added as much for decoration as for camouflage of pieced seams in the gray panels.

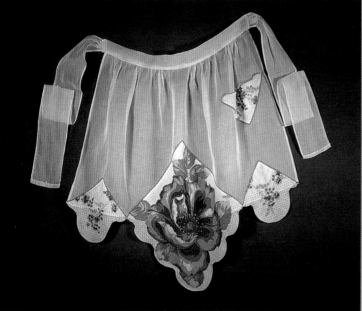

A magnificent floral handkerchief in **shades of purple and green** has been segmented and transformed into this lovely serving apron. A tiny dotted background and scalloped edges frame the flowers. The hanky sections are machine-stitched and complemented by the palest of pale lavender organdy. Miniature green rickrack highlights the lower edge and triangular pocket.

Lavender blooms and green foliage abound on this cotton percale apron. All seams and edges are neatly bound with lilac trim. A tumbler shaped patch pocket and a V-shaped waistband add suitable detailing to this **spacious four-sectioned apron**. And I mean *really* spacious. The apron measures 28 inches across at the waist, 60 inches across the lower edge, and 24 inches top to bottom.

You'll be **prepared for a royal event** in this organdy apron with its deep purple handkerchief pocket. Giant hibiscus-like flowers grace the set-on-point pocket, which is machine appliquéd to the apron. The waistline is lightly gathered and the sashes are pleated. The pocket is adjustable in fullness and shape with the 3/4-inch plastic ring.

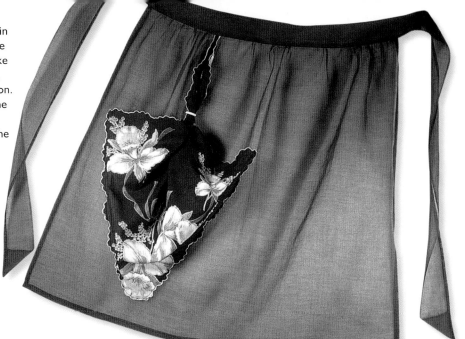

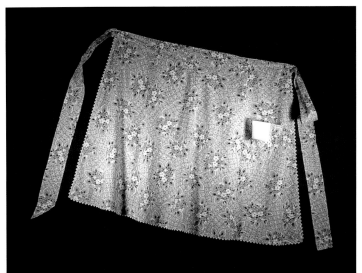

With an area of more than 840 square inches, this apron is among **the largest in the lot**. Enough for two or three separate aprons, some would say. The lovely lavender bouquet fabric is pieced in three sections and has lilac rickrack trim on the outer edges and center waist. The patch pocket is pretty well concealed.

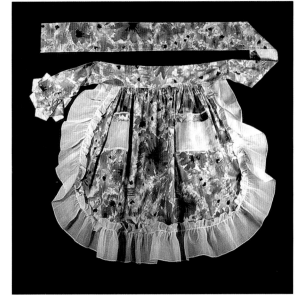

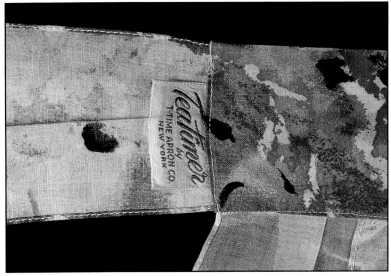

The **extremes of frivolity and practicality** can be seen in this and the next apron. Showy fabric, double ruffles, decorated organdy pockets, and generous sashes characterize this 'Teatimer' design. Thick gathers and a wide waistband top this rounded apron. A similar style of this apron can be found on page 51.

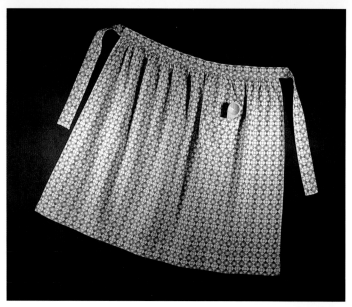

Abbreviated sashes and an absence of decoration characterize this practical apron. It is made from **a recycled feed sack** of a printed repeat design in lavender, blue, and green. Yes, there is a pocket. Can you spot the patched area (over a hole made from a weak spot in the original bag)?

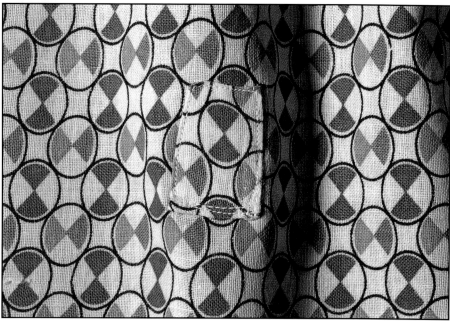

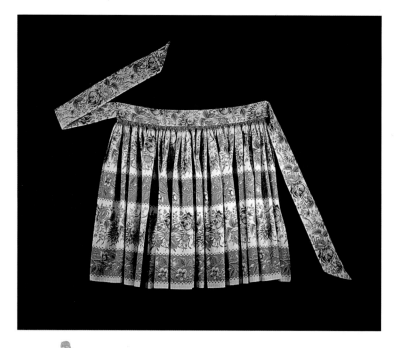

How many is **too many pleats?** How about 250 teensy-weensy ones? And that's not all. The lower edge measures seven feet in length. With a depth of seventeen inches, it is a massive amount of fabric for one apron. Numbers aside, one must admire the lovely lavender and rosy garlands in the border print cotton. Additional study of this apron shows that it was probably a commercially permanently pleated design whose pleats and permanence have worn out. The narrow vertical lines from pleating, pressing, and soil are just slightly visible. Another 'permanently pleated' apron (with pleats still intact) can be found in the *Seeing Red* section of this book.

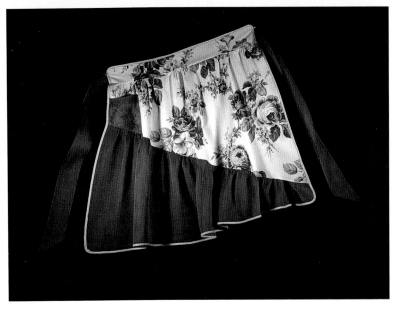

Surely among the most dramatic designs in this book, this ruffled and flowered apron could easily become the center of attention. The huge showy floral bouquets are complemented by the diagonally cut **deep purple organdy** skirt. Lime green bias edging provides an additional highlight. The odd-shaped organdy pocket has claimed a prominent position at top right.

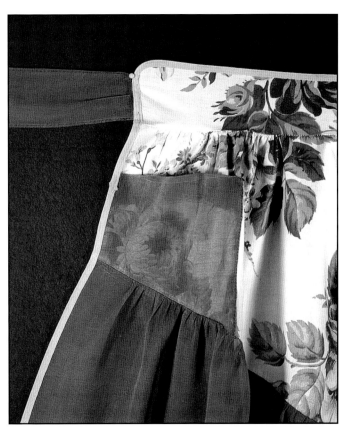

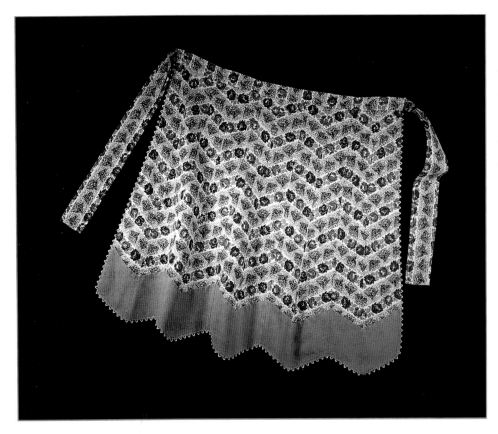

Purple and lilac flowers and a gray and black geometric pattern team up in this cotton percale fabric. Cut into **ten tapered gores** that are carefully matched and stitched into a subtle zigzag design, the apron is anchored with solid lilac cotton along the lower edge. An uncommon tricolor rickrack in green, white, and black edges the bottom and sides. What? No pocket?

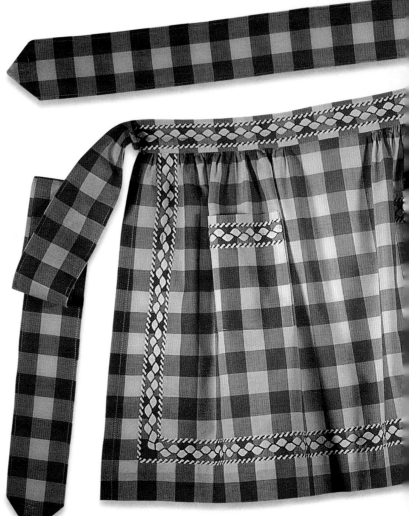

Several design details make this one inch lilac gingham apron a qualifier for **The Precision Award**: All rickrack detail is carefully placed along a single gingham line, the pockets are cut and placed to match the checks in the skirt, and the sashes are carefully cut along check lines (and mitered at the ends). All told, an impressive and eye-catching example of miniature and jumbo rickrack on jumbo gingham.

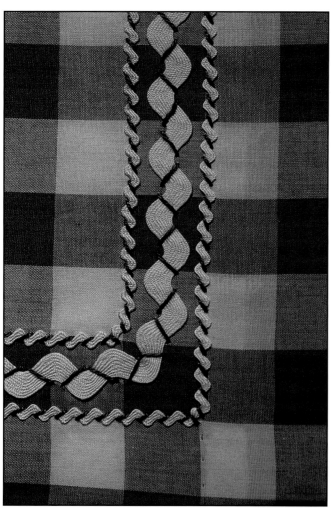

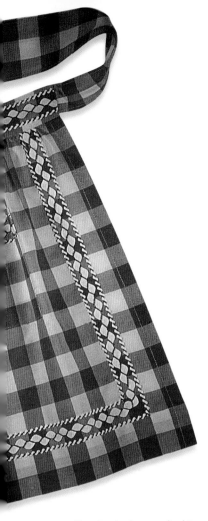

Purple gingham and white organdy make **the perfect combination** on this pleated half apron. Both small and large cross stitches are used in the stair step and border designs. White X's are stitched on the dark squares, forming eleven medallions framed in purple, and a decorative panel accents the waistband. A 'secret' pocket is cleverly placed on the right. From the collection of Betty Wilson.

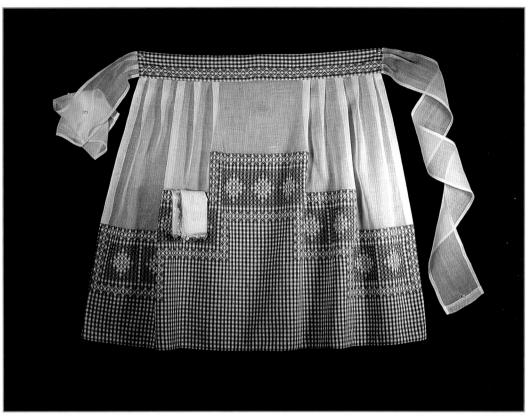

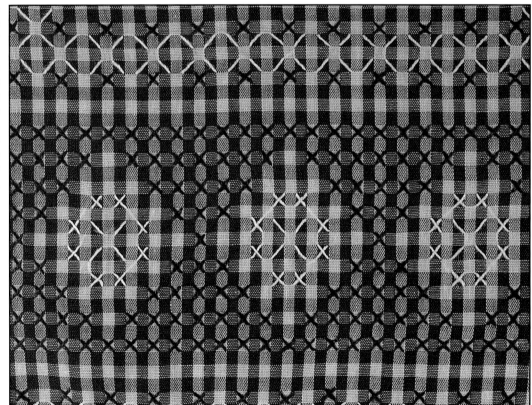

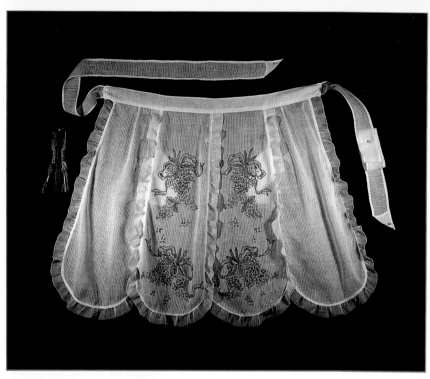

Generous **clusters of lilacs** form the centerpiece in this lightweight cotton apron. Shades of lavender and pale yellow are used in the flowers, which are further adorned with green foliage and orange ribbons and bows. One-inch wide sheer ruffles outline each of the four sections of the skirt. Can you detect the two hidden pockets?

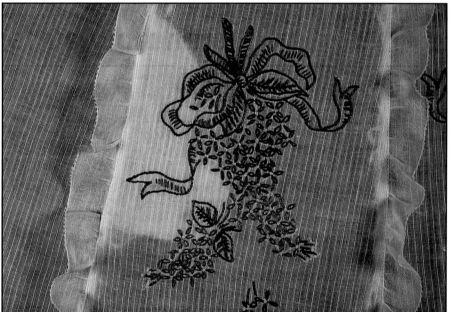

White shell braid with interwoven golden threads decorates this gathered apron. Strategically placed on the upper pocket, lower edge, and the ends of the sashes, it is a fine embellishment for the lightweight **translucent mauve** fabric. All trim has been hand applied. The extra long sashes are cut in one piece with the waistband.

Section Four

CHILDREN'S APRONS
(Plus Some for Grownups)

This may be the section to which you keep returning, for the sheer delight in viewing the aprons. Certainly these are among the most intriguing and alluring specimens in the apron world—for their diminutive nature, the cute and clever designs, and even the emotions and memories they may evoke.

If you wore an apron as a child, you will especially appreciate these designs—the efforts in their planning and construction, and the care and compassion associated with it. You may have your own treasured apron tucked away in the back of a closet, deep in a drawer, or retired in a cedar chest. If you no longer have the apron, you may at least have the cherished memory of it.

Three of the children's aprons in this section have a personal association for me. Two are from my family, ones that were made by my mother for my sister and me. A third apron is one that was worn by one of my children.

Several styles of children's aprons are included: Bibbed aprons, bibs, smocks, pinafores, and half aprons. Bibbed aprons can be identified by inclusion of a section to cover the upper part of the body. A bib is defined as: 1. "a cloth or plastic shield tied under a child's chin to protect the clothes;" or 2. "the part of an apron extending above the waist in the front". I would label an apron of the first definition a *bib*, an apron of the second definition a *bibbed apron*. I have taken the liberty of including some designs that more accurately should be labeled bibs (as opposed to bibbed aprons).

Smocks are a very common and extremely practical style for children's aprons (and also for adults). Generously cut to cover the entire upper body and a portion of the lower body, they may have a front or rear closure. Simply constructed and non-constrictive, they give liberal protection. They speak more of practicality, less of decoration.

Children's smocks may be associated as much with playtime and work time as with mealtime. Smocks for painting, gardening, or any home or school activities or tasks that require clothing protection are very common. Smocks for eating or helping Mom in the kitchen are a natural corollary.

A word to the wise about the difference between *smocks* and *smocking*: Smocks refer to the style of apron as described above; *smocking* refers to a needle art method of tucking used to embellish articles of clothing, including aprons. Two outstanding examples of smocking are included in this section—companion mother/daughter red gingham aprons. Two children's smocks are also included.

A pinafore is "a low-necked sleeveless apron, worn especially by children". The darlings of the children's aprons world, pinafores conjure up images of little girls in ruffles, ribbons, rickrack, and giant bows. In addition to the frills, pinafores have the basic apron components—a skirt, bib, sashes, and shoulder straps. Maybe even a pocket. Two superb examples of children's pinafore aprons are pictured.

Half aprons are the style of nearly every other apron described and pictured in this book. No bib, no shoulder or neck straps. Just the portion to cover the lower part of the front of the body (below the waist). They consist of a skirt, a waistband (usually), sashes, and perhaps a pocket. Several examples are pictured, including designs with rickrack, cross stitch, smocking, pleating, and an ever-so-tiny turquoise gingham checked apron for a child.

And just where would you look to find children's aprons? Among the most highly valued by dealers and cherished by owners, they are the most difficult to find. The best sources may be family, friends, and per-

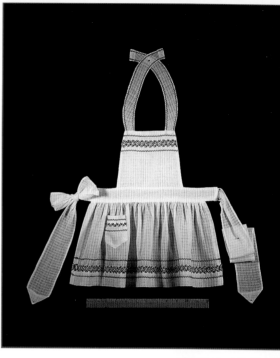

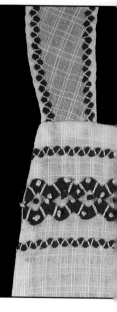

Scarlet rickrack joins with lightweight white windowpane cotton in this exquisite **child's pinafore apron**. Generous sashes and gently curved shoulder straps are attached to the waistband and bodice. Paired rows of miniature and regular rickrack are stitched with white embroidery thread and decorated with French knots in contrasting colors. Made by Lena Voss, from the collection of Arda Davis.

sonal acquaintances. Many remain in private collections, just because of their emotional attachment. For most children's aprons owners, treasured memories carry more weight than monetary value.

The next best place to look for children's aprons, after your own closets, and those of your family and friends, is at garage sales and flea markets. Once in a while they make their way to a thrift sale table or a dealer's stall. Inevitably you will find children's aprons at antique malls and stores. They are usually prominently displayed and prohibitively priced. But sometimes you can get lucky and find one by rummaging in the bottom of a drawer, bin, or basket full of jumbled and rumpled miscellaneous linens.

Just how do we determine that an apron is really a *child's* apron? Some are obviously so, based on dimensions (small size) or proportions (miniaturized). Some have juvenile design elements such as animals, toys, letters, and numbers (not a sure indication, as similar juvenile themes are sometimes found on adult aprons!). Sometimes it is difficult to know. Two of the half-aprons included in this section may not have been intended for children. They are included because they have uncharacteristically small dimensions. They may have been intended for large children; or perhaps for small adults.

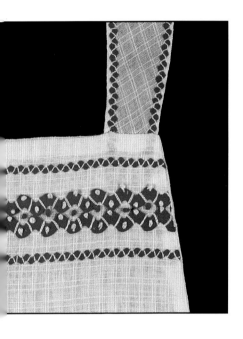

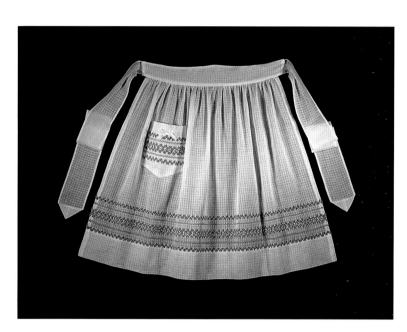

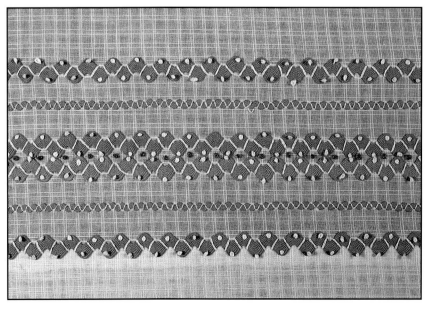

And here's the **companion apron for Mom**. Similarly hand constructed from lightweight cotton, this lightly gathered half apron also features a shaped waistband and yards of copen blue rickrack. A white satin ribbon bow tops the five-sided pocket. All stitching is done by hand. Made by Lena Voss, from the collection of Arda Davis.

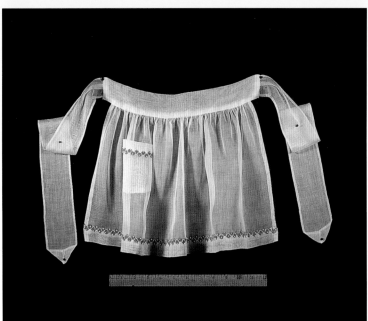

Bright pink rickrack takes the limelight on this sheer organdy pale pink apron. Most remarkable is the **exquisite handwork**. Everything is done by hand—hemming, gathering, and appliqué work. The rickrack trim is attached with decorative stitches and French knots worked in double-stranded white embroidery floss. Made by Lena Voss, from the collection of Arda Davis.

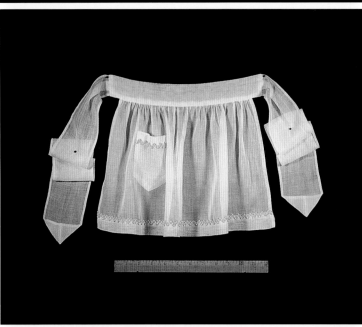

This airy yellow gathered apron is the companion for the preceding design. It is similarly embellished with **turquoise rickrack** on the pocket and along the lower edge. The pentagonal pocket is secured with tiny appliqué stitches. Made by Lena Voss, from the collection of Arda Davis.

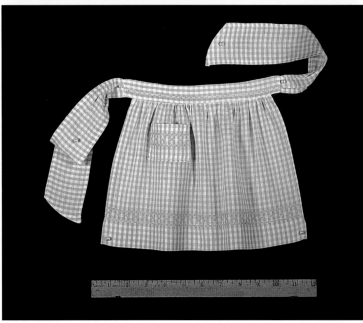

Surely among **the smallest of gingham aprons**, this child's version measures a mere 7 1/2 inches deep and a scant 13 inches wide. Tiny cross stitches decorate the lower edge, waistband, and miniature pocket. Sash ends are gently rounded. The box style pleats on the sashes are placed one in and one out.

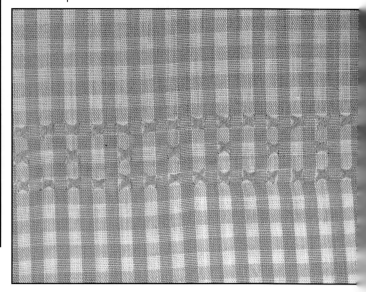

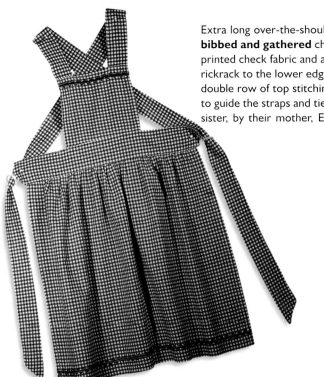

Extra long over-the-shoulder straps are among the requirements for this **bibbed and gathered** child's apron. Also about a half yard of blue and white printed check fabric and a package of lipstick-red rickrack. Attach the rickrack to the lower edge of the skirt and the upper edge of the bib with a double row of top stitching in white thread. You'll also need two plastic rings to guide the straps and tie the bow at the back. Made for the author and her sister, by their mother, Eilene Paulson.

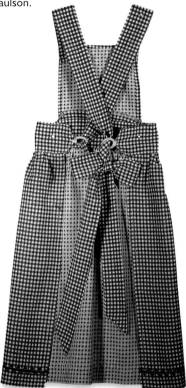

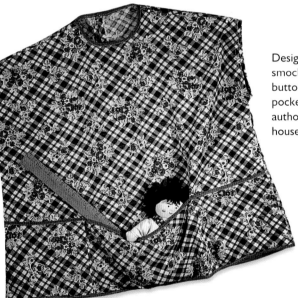

Designed and constructed with **a child's needs** in mind, this practical smock has three pockets. A rear button closure has hand worked buttonholes, and the perimeter of the neckline, lower edge, and pockets are bound with pink bias tape. This smock was made for the author and her sister, by their mother, Eilene Paulson. (She also made a housecoat for herself in the 1950s, from the same fabric.)

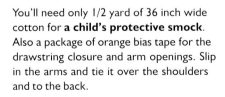

You'll need only 1/2 yard of 36 inch wide cotton for **a child's protective smock**. Also a package of orange bias tape for the drawstring closure and arm openings. Slip in the arms and tie it over the shoulders and to the back.

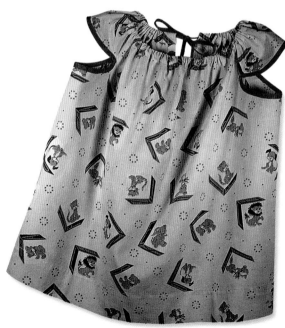

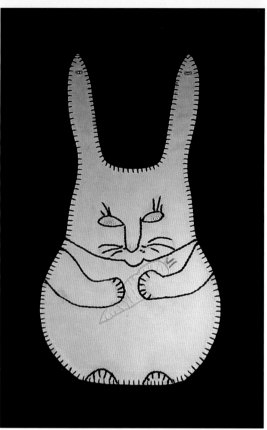

This **long-eared, carrot-munching, bottom-heavy bunny** would delight any child. Technically not an apron, but rather a bib, it is made from cotton percale and is fully lined. Details are hand embroidered stem stitches using six strands of floss in black, pink, and yellow. The edges are outlined with black blanket stitches. There is no evidence of a closure at the neckline (snaps, hook and eye, or ties might have been appropriate). Perhaps a pin was used.

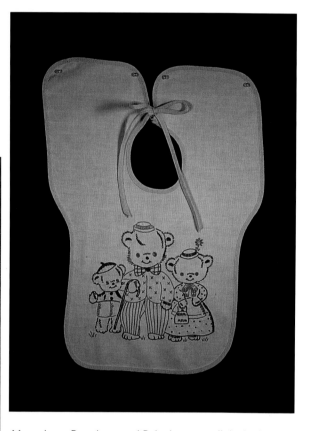

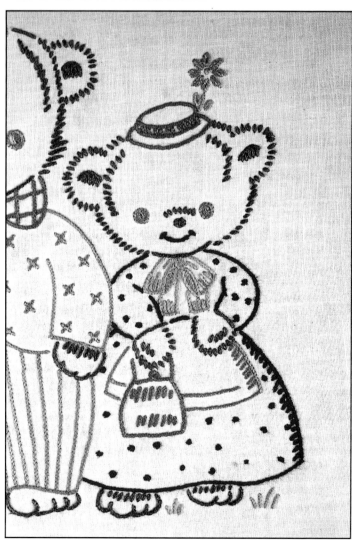

Mama bear, Papa bear, and Baby bear are all decked out with bow tie, purse, cane, and hats on this one-piece cotton bib. All details on the **three smiling brown bears** are neatly embroidered in red, orange, blue, and green. The edges are finished with pale yellow bias trim, which transforms naturally into the ties.

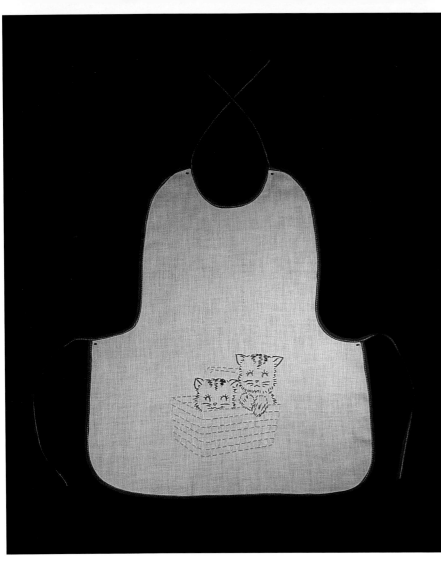

Two **cute and curious kittens** are peeking from the embroidered basket of this child's unbleached cotton muslin apron. Large running stitches in gold thread form the basket; stem stitches in two shades of brown define the kittens. Bright red narrow bias trim is used for the ties at the neck and waist, as well as the outer edges.

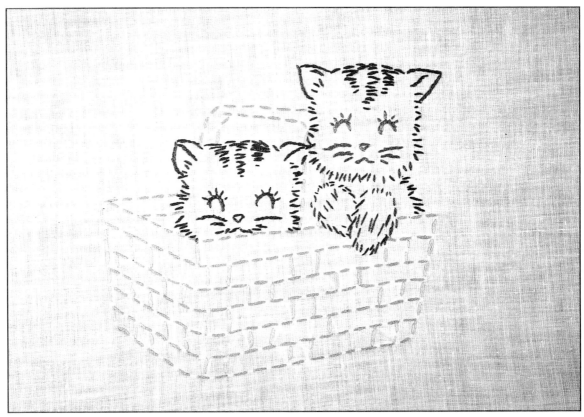

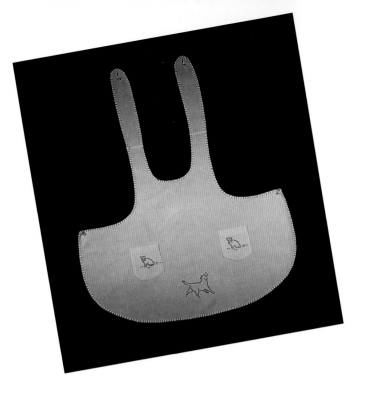

This clever arrangement of over-the-shoulder straps that cross over and button to the back of this cotton percale apron would provide **ample coverage** for any child. A playful puppy is embroidered on the lower front, and companion kittens decorate the twin pockets. All outer edges are hemmed and embroidered with sky blue blanket stitches. The buttons are 3/8-inch pearl and the buttonholes are handworked.

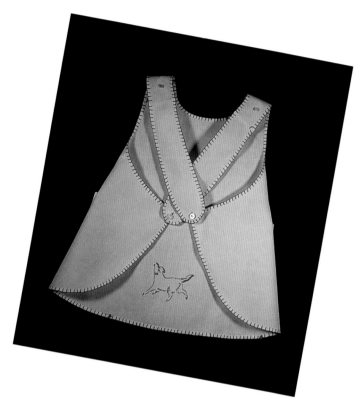

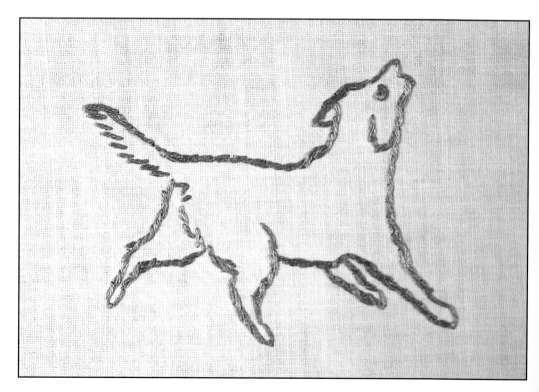

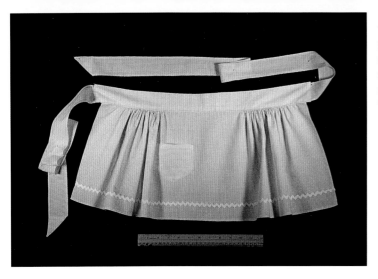

This printed mini-checked buttercup yellow apron is only 10 inches deep, but it has **72 inches of sash**. Perhaps it's for a short not-so-thin person. Even the lower edge of the apron measures a full 36 inches, as if the maker were taking full advantage of the cross width of the fabric. Details include a five-sided pocket and white rickrack trim.

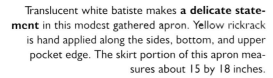

Translucent white batiste makes **a delicate statement** in this modest gathered apron. Yellow rickrack is hand applied along the sides, bottom, and upper pocket edge. The skirt portion of this apron measures about 15 by 18 inches.

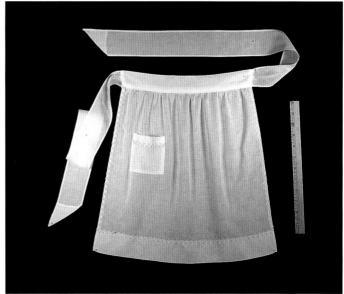

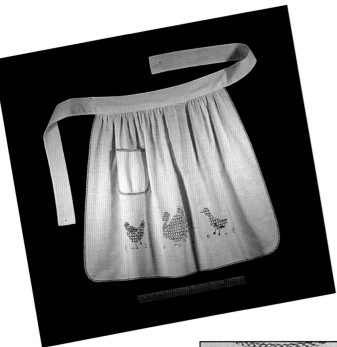

Loosely woven unbleached cotton muslin serves as the background for the cross stitched rooster, turkey, and duck on this child's apron. Made from a prestamped commercial kit, the embroidery was rendered **by a child, for a child**. Tiny hand-stitched flowers and golden stalks of grain surround the birds, and red checked bias trim accents the rounded pocket and lower edges. Apron made by and from the collection of Virginia Bregel.

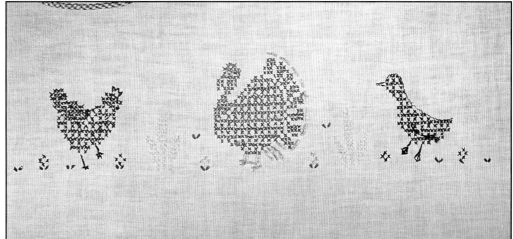

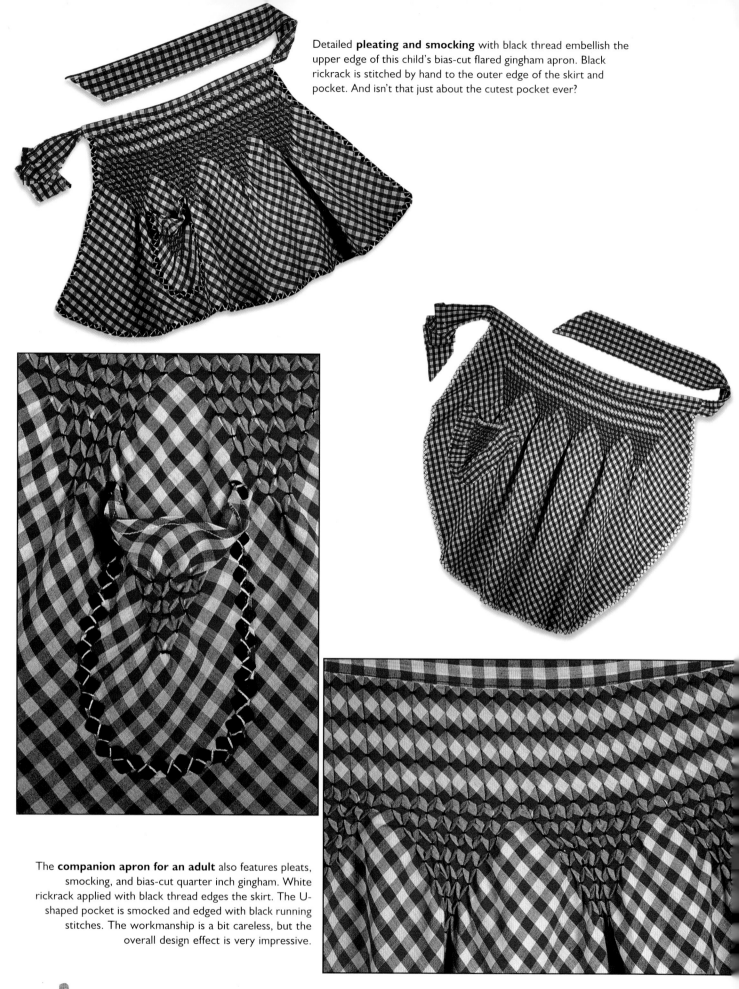

Detailed **pleating and smocking** with black thread embellish the upper edge of this child's bias-cut flared gingham apron. Black rickrack is stitched by hand to the outer edge of the skirt and pocket. And isn't that just about the cutest pocket ever?

The **companion apron for an adult** also features pleats, smocking, and bias-cut quarter inch gingham. White rickrack applied with black thread edges the skirt. The U-shaped pocket is smocked and edged with black running stitches. The workmanship is a bit careless, but the overall design effect is very impressive.

Appendix:
An Assortment of Vintage
Apron Patterns & Kits

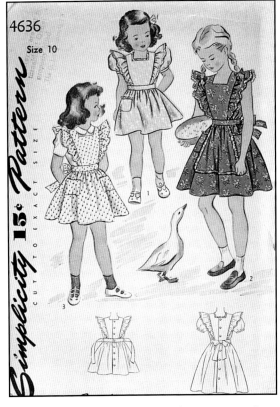

Simplicity #4636, 15¢ (unprinted pattern pieces)

Many pattern companies printed and sold apron patterns during the 20th century. Simplicity, McCall's, Butterick, and Advance produced a variety of designs in the 1930s, 1940s, and 1950s. Other companies published patterns and made them available through mail order advertisements, a common method for procuring patterns.

Apron patterns were also available in kit form. Packages typically included the prestamped fabric for the apron, threads, special trimmings, and instructions. The apron might be completely preassembled, requiring only the decorative stitching and embellishments, or it might require both assembly and decoration. Examples of two apron needlework kits are shown.

Twenty-five vintage apron printed patterns are featured in this appendix. The name of the company, pattern number, date, and price for each pattern are included, if known. Several patterns have unprinted pieces, suggesting a pre-1940s publication. The lower prices also suggest an early printing date. Descriptions and additional details about instructions, pieces, package contents, or mail order sources are noted for some patterns.

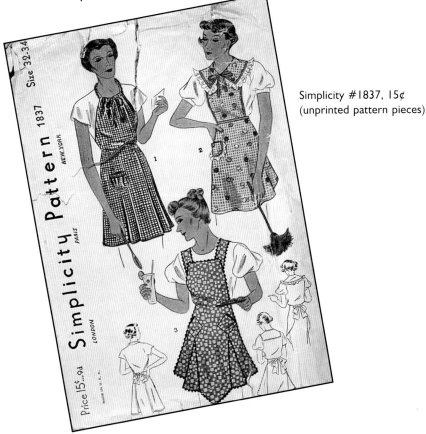

Simplicity #1837, 15¢
(unprinted pattern pieces)

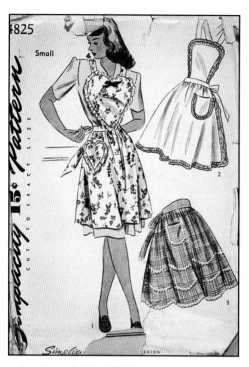

Simplicity #4825, ©1943, 15¢

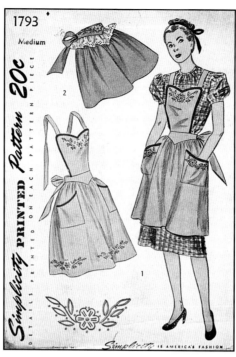

Simplicity #1793, ©1946, 20¢

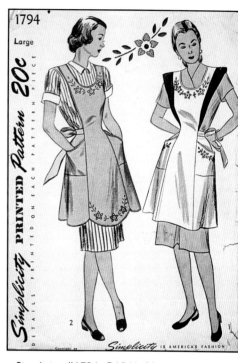

Simplicity #1794, ©1946, 20¢

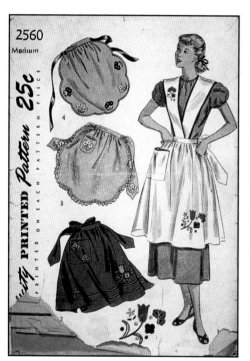

Simplicity #2560, ©1946, 25¢

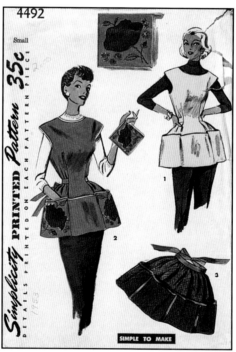

Simplicity #4492, ©1953, 35¢

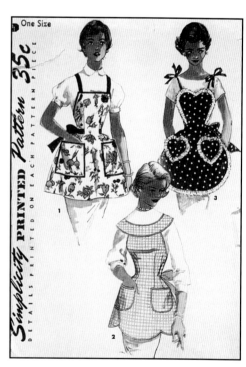

Simplicity #1359, ©1955, 35¢

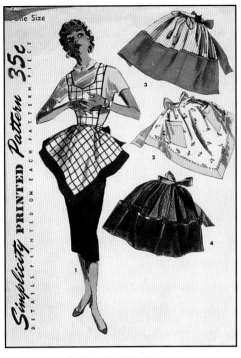

Simplicity #1391, ©1955, 35¢

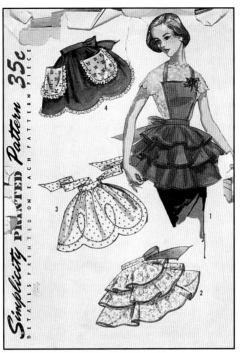

Simplicity #1805, ©1956, 35¢

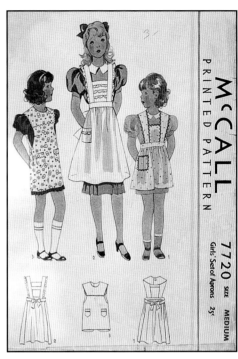

McCall's #7720, ©1934, 25¢

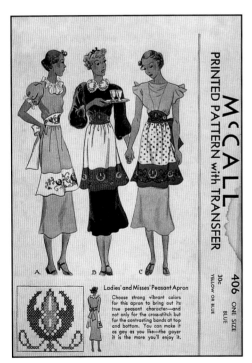

McCall's #406, ©1936, 30¢

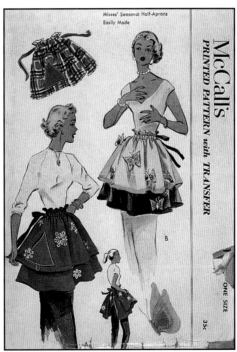

McCall's #1714, ©1952, 35¢

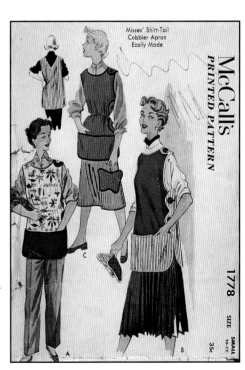

McCall's #1778, ©1953, 35¢

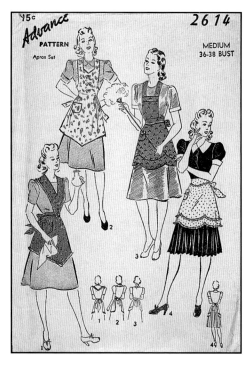

Advance #2614, 15¢ (unprinted pattern pieces)

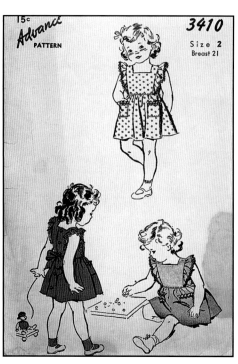

Advance #3410, 15¢ (unprinted pattern pieces)

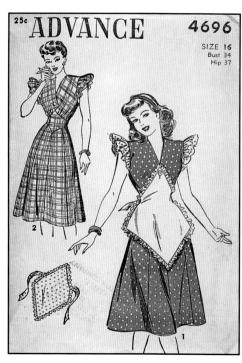

Advance #4696, 25¢

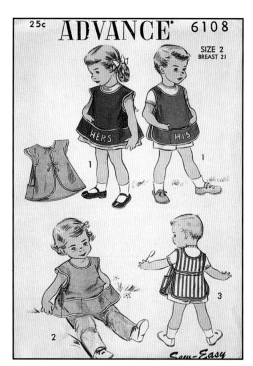

Advance #6108, 25¢ (unprinted pattern pieces)

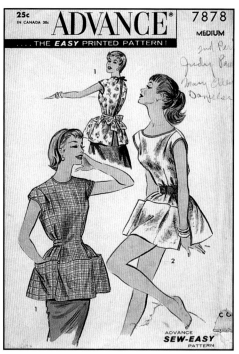

Advance #7878, 25¢ (This pattern was used by the author during her 1959-60 freshman home economics class. Her apron is pictured in the Introduction of this book.)

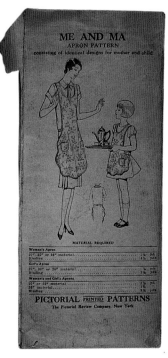

Pictorial Review Company, "Me and Ma" apron pattern, ©1925

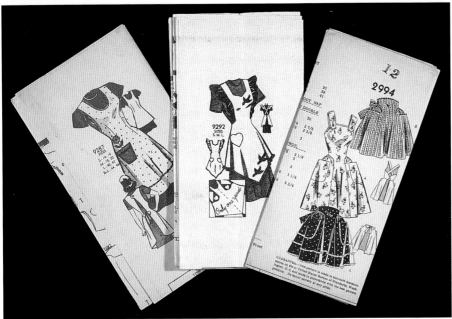

Marian Martin #9287 (ordered through Dairyland News Pattern Department, Lake Mills, WI, postage 1½ ¢); Marian Martin #9292 (ordered through Pattern Department, New York); Fashion Service #2994 (ordered through The Pattern Bureau, New York)

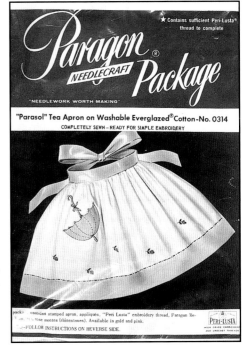

Paragon® Needlecraft Package No. 0314, "Parasol" Tea Apron on Washable Everglazed® Cotton (completely sewn—ready for simple embroidery)

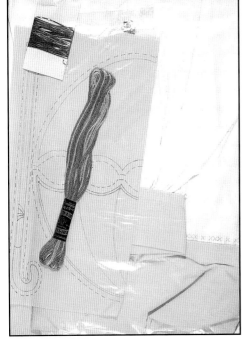

Paragon® Needlecraft Package No. 0314 (rear view)

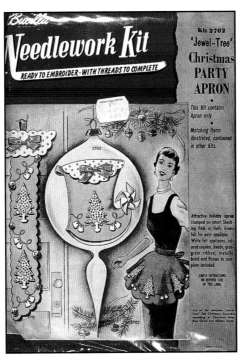

Bucilla® "do-it-yourself" Needlework Kit, Kit 2702 "Jewel-Tree" Christmas Party Apron, $2.25, (ready to embroider—with threads to complete)

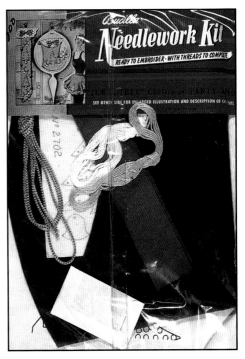

Bucilla® "do-it-yourself" Needlework Kit, Kit 2702 (rear view)

A Word About Values

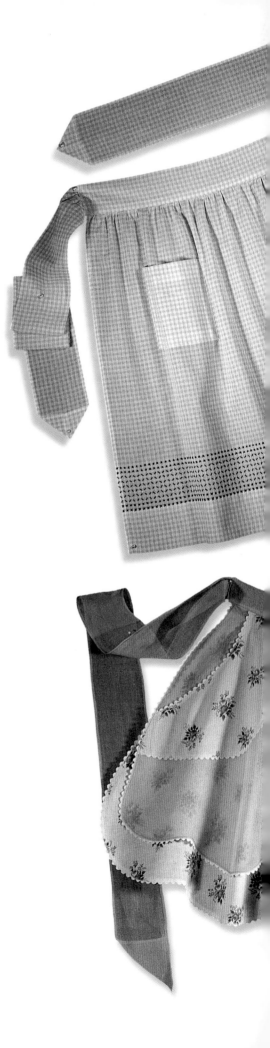

The fast growing popularity of vintage textiles and the sentimentality of the mid-20th century has brought long overdue attention to the world of apron collecting. Because the textiles and linens market remains disorganized, real values are often unrecognized. However, both avid and novice collectors and a generation of baby boomers drawn to the nostalgia of the 1930s-1960s are now witnessing a steady climb in the value of once largely-ignored items like the American apron.

The 200 aprons in this collection are not individually valued. However, I can make several helpful observations and comments. First, I prefer a value guide, as opposed to a price guide. Because the majority of aprons from my collection (and perhaps yours, too) were found in garage sales, flea markets, and resale shops, they were mostly under-priced, and the specific dollar amounts paid are less useful in this instance. To divulge exactly how much I paid for specific aprons would be of little help to the reader.

Many value guides use a simple graduated scale based on the condition of the item (a scale of say four or five categories such as mint, excellent, very good, good, fair, or poor), condition being based on presence and amount of damage, defects, and anything that distracts from the perfection of the item. In the case of aprons, these might be such things as holes, tears, stains, deterioration, general wear and tear, and noticeable flaws. (Yes, fabric has flaws, too.) Although the presence of such 'distractions' would customarily detract from the apron and reduce its monetary value, some collectors (myself included) might consider such 'flaws' as attractive design features. A skillfully repaired hole in a recycled feed sack apron will look like a 'worn and mended garment' to most viewers. To others, it is a carefully hand stitched miniature work of art that reflects the flavor and frugality of an era. Although it may be presumptuous to elevate a mended apron to the level of textile art, we do know that the beauty of the fabric alone may qualify it. And, heaven knows, in our modern throwaway culture, meticulous hand mending may in itself be collectible.

Another system of evaluation for linens and textiles involves the use of stars, one to five, to measure 'collectibility': one star is collectible, two stars is very collectible, three stars is highly collectible, four stars is extremely collectible, and five stars is most collectible. This system may be more useful in the emerging textiles market. Similar to a system of rating fine (and not-so-fine) restaurants or movies, I personally use a star system to rate books I have read. It has its drawbacks. What I consider collectible (and in the case of books, which ones I would enthusiastically recommend or not recommend at all) is highly personal and subjective.

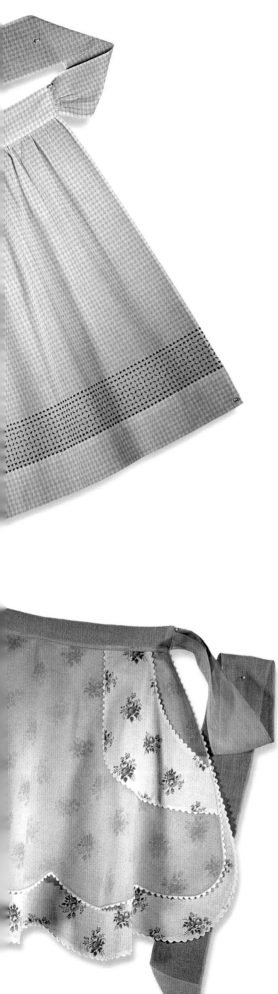

The over-riding factor in what ends up in my apron collection is whether I like it or not. What is 'highly collectible' to me is perhaps of little value or worthless to others. So you will find no descriptive words (mint, excellent, etc.), stars (* to *****), or dollar amounts assigned to the aprons in this book.

Nevertheless, it is important and beneficial to understand what factors determine the price of an apron at an antique shop or collectibles market. Many of these detailed factors are difficult or impossible to ascertain, as many aprons are handmade and produced in the home, while others are factory made and store bought. Take the following items into consideration:

1. Date or age of apron (often difficult to determine)
2. Condition (wear, stains, holes)
3. Size (half apron, full apron)
4. Style (smock, cobbler, children's)
5. Hand needlework (amount and kind)
6. Fabrics and fibers (natural, synthetic)
7. Regional demand

I have paid more than twenty-five dollars ($25) for a meticulously and entirely hand stitched red and white cross stitched and rickracked gingham apron in excellent condition. I have also paid nine cents (yes, 9¢) for another red and white gingham apron. More importantly, I would have willingly paid considerably more for the second apron because it was an unusual half-inch gingham which I have had difficulty finding. For me, it carried a great deal of value.

Keeping in mind that aprons are a relatively new area of interest, they are mostly undervalued, prices are speculative, and tastes vary widely, the following value guide may be helpful:

Valued at less than $10:
Synthetic fabrics and blends
Poorly constructed aprons (home made or store bought)

Valued at $10 to $25:
Factory made half aprons
Ordinary gingham aprons with minimal cross stitching or rickrack
Handkerchief aprons

Valued at $25 to $50:
Entirely hand sewn aprons
Aprons embellished with hand embroidery or crochet
Appliquéd and pieced aprons

Valued at $50 or more:
Aprons from the 19th or early 20th century
Children's aprons
Aprons with intricate hand needlework (lace, tatting)

Glossary

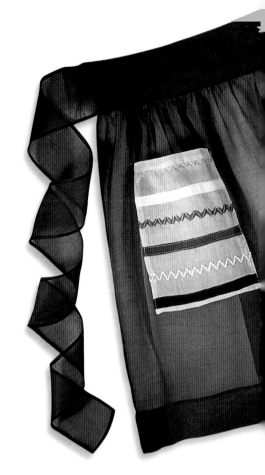

appliqué: An ornamentation, as for cloth, cut from one material and laid down upon another.

apron: A garment, usually of cloth, plastic, or leather usually tied onto the front of the body with strings around the waist and used to protect clothing or adorn a costume. (Etymology: Middle English alteration of *napron* from Middle French *naperon*, diminutive of *nape* cloth, modification of Latin *mappa* napkin.)

batiste: (French) General term for soft, lightweight thin fabric made in a plain weave of cotton or synthetic fibers such as rayon. Used for dresses, blouses, handkerchiefs, and infants' wear. Batiste is the finest and softest of the related plain weave cloths such as lawn.

bib: A cloth or plastic shield tied under a child's chin to protect the clothes; the part of an apron extending above the waist in the front.

broadcloth: Term used to describe several dissimilar fabrics made with different fibers, weaves, and finishes; cotton broadcloth is a fine fabric with a slight rib in the filling direction.

complementary (colors): Relating to or constituting one of a pair of contrasting colors that produce a neutral color when combined in suitable proportions; opposite on the color wheel.

cross stitch: Basic X-shaped stitches applied to mesh or fabric; a common embellishment stitch on gingham aprons.

dotted organdy or dotted Swiss: Sheer, crisp, plain weave nylon or cotton organdy permanently flocked with evenly spaced, raised dots.

Empire: Characteristic of costume during the French Empire period (1804-14); marked by high waistline; in a skirt, cut to extend from two to four inches above normal waistline.

flocking (or flocked): A fabric is first printed with an adhesive, then dusted with short fibers (flocks) which adhere to the adhesive, forming a design that stands in relief to the surface of the fabric.

floweret (floret): A small flower, especially one of the small flowers forming the head of a composite plant.

gingham: (Malay *gingan*) A cotton cloth, usually in stripes or checks, of two or more colors, woven of dyed yarn, and used for dresses, aprons, etc.

gore: A tapering or triangular piece used to give a varying width (as of cloth in a skirt).

grosgrain: A silk or rayon fabric (or ribbon) with crosswise cotton ribs.

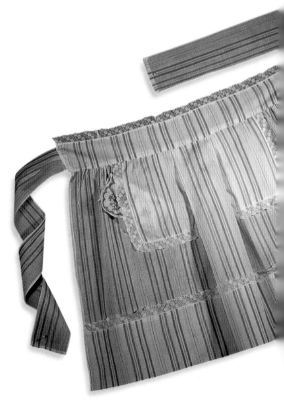

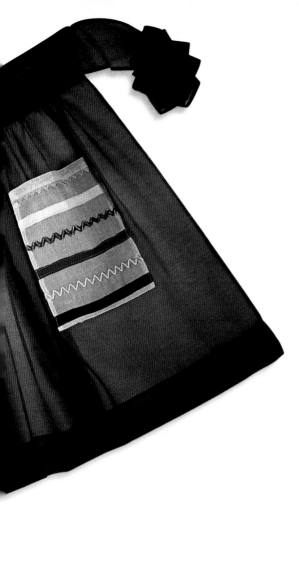

handkerchief: A small usually square piece of cloth used for various usually personal purposes or as a costume accessory.

huck: Short for huckaback, absorbent cotton or linen toweling fabric of figured weave, with prominent weft threads. Used for towels, fancy work.

kitsch: Artistic or literary material of low quality.

lawn: Lightweight, sheer, fine cotton or linen fabric. May be given a soft or crisp finish. It is treated to give it a soft, lustrous appearance.

linen: A cloth made of flax and noted for its strength, coolness, and luster.

linens: Clothing or household articles made of linen cloth or similar fabric.

mercerized: Cotton thread or fabric treated with caustic alkali (sodium hydroxide) so that it is strengthened, made more receptive of dyes, and given a silken sheen.

muslin: Term for a large group of plain weave cotton fabrics ranging from light to heavy; may be bleached, unbleached, or printed.

organdy (organdie): A sheer, lightweight, plain weave fabric of cotton, silk, or synthetic fiber with a rather stiff wiry feel. The yarns are fine, the weave fairly open. Some finishes may be applied.

organza: Similar to organdy, but more wiry and transparent. Made of silk or synthetic fiber yarns. The yarns are highly twisted.

ornamentation: The addition of something that lends grace and beauty; adornment.

percale: Firm, smooth, plain weave cotton fabric that is starched and has little luster.

pinafore: A low-necked sleeveless apron worn especially by children.

pulled thread: Also known as drawn work; a method of removal of threads (horizontal or vertical) creating an open space in which remaining threads may be grouped and secured, or into which new embroidery or lace designs may be inserted.

reversible: Having two finished usable sides; wearable with either side out.

rickrack (or ricrac): A flat braid woven to form zigzags and used especially as trimming for clothing.

selvage (selvedge): The edge on either side of a fabric so finished as to prevent raveling.

smock: An overgarment of washable material used, especially by women and children, to protect the clothes.

smocking: A decorative embroidery or shirring made by gathering cloth in regularly spaced round tucks.

Swedish (huck) weaving: A decorative arrangement of spaced running embroidery stitches on huck (huckaback) toweling, which has small raised loops which occur at regular intervals, used for darning the designs. Also used on dotted organdy fabric.

taffeta: A crisp plain-woven lustrous fabric of various fibers, used especially for women's clothing.

tatting: A delicate handmade lace formed usually by looping and knotting with a single cotton thread and a small shuttle.

Teneriffe lace (traditional): A lace made using a blunt needle and smooth thread, with darning and knotting stitches over a web of threads stretched across a small pinwheel, to form a medallion. Also known as wheel lace.

tulle: (from the town Tulle, France) A fine lightweight small hexagonal mesh net fabric.

turquoise: A variable color averaging a light greenish blue, very popular in the 1950s and 1960s.

References

Advance Pattern Co., Inc. Printed Patterns #2614, #3410, #4696, #6108, and #7878. New York: Advance Pattern Co., Inc.

Bell, Louise Price. *Kitchen Fun - A Cook Book for Children*. Cleveland: The Harter Publishing Company, 1932.

Betty Crocker's Cook Book for Boys and Girls. Illustrated by Gloria Kamen. New York: Golden Press, 1957.

Clothing Fabrics - Facts for Consumer Education. Home Economics Research Report No. 1. United States Department of Agriculture, Issued April 1957.

Electric Cooking with your Hotpoint Automatic Range. Chicago: Hotpoint Institute.

The Elson Pupil's Hand Chart. Chicago, Atlanta, and New York: Scott, Foresman and Company, 1937.

Learn How Book - Coats & Clark's Book No. 170-B. New York: Coats & Clark's Sales Corp., 1959.

Manchester, Marsha. *Vintage White Linens A to Z*. Atglen, PA: Schiffer Publishing Ltd., 1997.

Mary Alden's Cookbook for Children - Easy Step-by-step Picture Recipes in Full Color. Pictures by Dorothy King. New York: Wonder Books, Inc., 1955.

McCall Corporation. Printed Patterns #7720, #406, #1714, and #1778. The McCall Corporation, 1934-53.

Montgomery Ward. 1942-43 Fall/Winter Catalog. St. Paul, MN.

Montgomery Ward. 1971 Fall/Winter Catalog. St. Paul, MN.

National Cotton Council. *How to Sew and Save with Cotton Bags*.

O'Neill, Mary. *Hailstones & Halibut Bones*. New York: Doubleday & Co., Inc., 1961.

Picken, Mary Brooks. *The Fashion Dictionary - Fabric, Sewing, and Dress as expressed in the Language of Fashion*. New York: Funk & Wagnalls Company, 1957.

Recipe and Instruction Book - Hamilton Beach Mixette. Racine, WI: Hamilton Beach Company (Division, Scovill Manufacturing Co.).

Scofield, Elizabeth, and Peggy Zalamea. *20th Century Linens and Lace - A Guide to Identification, Care, and Prices of Household Linens*. Atglen, PA: Schiffer Publishing Ltd., 1995.

Sears, Roebuck and Co. 1922 Catalog. Minneapolis, MN.

Sears, Roebuck and Co. 1935-36 Fall/Winter Catalog. Minneapolis, MN.

Simplicity Pattern Co., Inc. Printed Patterns #1359, #1391, #1793, #1794, #1805, #1837, #2560, #4492, #4636, and #4825. New York: Simplicity Pattern Co., Inc., 1943-56.

Simplicity Sewing Book - Easy Guide for Beginners and Experts. New York: Simplicity Pattern Co. Inc., 1954.

Stillwell, Alexandra. *The Techniques of Teneriffe Lace*. Watertown, MA: Charles T. Branford Co., 1980.

Textile Handbook (Fourth Edition). Washington D.C.: American Home Economics Association, 1970.

Westinghouse Home Economics Institute. *Home Laundering Guide for Clothes and Fabrics*. Mansfield, OH: Westinghouse Electric & Mfg. Co., 1944.

Wright, Roxa, assisted by Margot Knox. *How to Make Aprons*. New York: M. Barrows and Company, Inc., 1953.

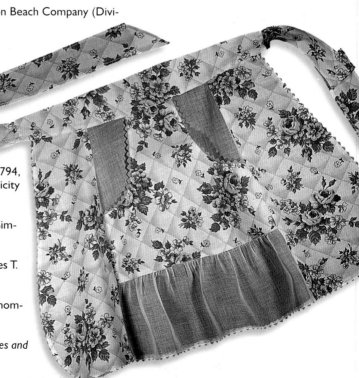